Aim for Success Parent Presentation

Why Encourage Sexual Abstinence

1. Pregnancy

2. Sexually Transmitted Diseases

3. Emotional Scars

4. Failure Rates of Condoms

5. How Far is too Far

6. Dangers of Alcohol and Drug Use

When and How to Encourage Sexual Abstinence

1. Teach your children your values

2. Be there for your children

3. Give your children lots of love

Aim for Success, Inc. is one of the largest providers of sexual abstinence education in the nation. This non-profit, educational organization has appeared in *Time* and *World* magazines and on Fox News-New York. They have received recognition from Focus on the Family, First Lady Nancy Reagan, and Texas Governor George W. Bush.

Aim for Success, Inc. • **P.O. Box 550336** • **Dallas, Texas 75355**
(972) 422-2322 • **Fax: (972) 422-8030**
www.aimforsuccess.org • **Email: office@aimforsuccess.org**

A B C's

of the Birds and Bees

for Parents of Toddlers to Teens

A B C's

of the Birds and Bees

for Parents of Toddlers to Teens

By

Marilyn Morris

CHARLES RIVER PUBLISHING COMPANY

Dallas, Texas

A B C's
of the Birds and Bees
for Parents of Toddlers to Teens

Written by Marilyn Morris

Cover by Charles Joseph
Illustrations by Shannan McEowen

PRINTING HISTORY
First Edition: 1999
Second Edition: 2000

ISBN: 0-9648113-5-9
Library of Congress Card Number: 99-091875

For information address:

Charles River Publishing Company
P.O. Box 551623
Dallas, TX 75355

PRINTED IN THE UNITED STATES OF AMERICA

ACKNOWLEDGEMENTS

To Chuck, my husband and best friend,
who inspired, encouraged, and supported
me through every step of this project.

Special thanks to the following men who provided invaluable
assistance in the research and development of this book:

William Fackler, M.D.
Joe McIlhaney, M.D.
Richard Tompkins, Ph.D.
Hal Wallis, M.D.
Paul Warren, M.D.

Life and sex are both precious gifts from God entrusted to the family. Procreation literally gives life to children and families. Accurate teaching about the basics of life – including sex and sexuality – imparts knowledge and promotes maturity. This is always most effective and meaningful when it takes place within the family. *This book is about life, sex and the family.*

Truth brings freedom to life through encouraging proper life choices. Ignorance, misconceptions, and lies lead to poor life choices, bringing bondage to human life. Our culture has witnessed the devastation of sexual immorality stemming from the avoidance of truth about sexuality. The quality of life as well as life itself are threatened. *This book is about truth.*

Character is the result of life application of truth, through wise but often tough life choices. Character is a critical source of self esteem and an essential part of healthy sexuality. Character is best taught to children and teenagers through strong, nurturing family relationships. *This book is about families and character.*

Drawing from her own life experiences and her passion for the quality of life, Marilyn Morris brings a contagious enthusiasm to her challenge to families to celebrate the gift of life by becoming sexually educated and character strengthened. This book presents the choice of abstinence outside of marriage as the only way to restore the joy of sex. *This book is about choices that lead to lifelong success.*

Paul A. Warren, MD

Dr. Warren is a behavioral pediatrician, author,
and respected international speaker.

The last two decades have seen the world regarding sexuality undergo phenomenal changes. When I began practicing Gynecology in the late 1970s, no one would have predicted that we would be in the midst of a pandemic of sexually transmitted diseases (STDs) by the mid-1990s. We find ourselves in just that position, with the spread of bacterial and viral diseases in unprecedented proportions worldwide. The message that limited sexual contact and condom usage would prevent the very epidemic in which we find ourselves has proven to be an utter failure. Literally, billions of dollars have been spent in an attempt to educate two generations of young people about the dangers of STDs, but we have found that education about the mechanics of sexuality is not enough to prevent the consequences of poor behavior.

The world shows us through the media and through the promotion of lackadaisical sexual attitudes that sexuality is a toy to be brought out and played with then put away for future enjoyment with no consequences. We never see the movie star in the emergency room with a ruptured ectopic pregnancy or undergoing surgery for complications of Human Papilloma Virus (now the most common STD). Yet these are true-life results of the policies and attitudes that treat sexuality in such a flippant way.

Our children deserve to know the whole truth about sexuality and its inherent dangers and joys. We condemn a generation of young people to failure when we say 'they are going to do it anyway' and treat them as if they have no consciences and no ability to weigh the dangers of their actions.

Marilyn Morris is one of only a handful who has been willing to step to the table and present the whole story of human sexuality, both the good and the bad. As a physician I have long recognized that a mechanistic approach to teaching sexuality, which ignored the psychosocial ramifications to the individual, the family, and society, was doomed to failure. Only a comprehensive approach such as the one presented in this work will offer any real hope that we may convince this generation of adolescents that their sexual relationships are to be treasured. It is in seeking this special relationship with one other individual that the true meaning of sexuality in our lives may reach its full potential.

It is my hope that families who use this tool will not only be blessed as they seek to fulfill their own hopes and dreams, but that through this parent-child dialogue, our society will reap the benefits as human sexuality regains its proper place and perspective.

Hal Wallis, MD
Fellow, American College of OB-GYN
Chair, Texas Physician Resource Council

TABLE OF CONTENTS

Introduction

As parents we all want the best for our children. It seems the universal goal all parents have for their children is a long, successful life with a minimum of pain and difficulties.

Today, one of the most prevalent problems afflicting our children, causing serious pain and difficulties, is the consequence of sex. We all seem to know someone who had to quit school because of a pregnancy or parents who are raising their grandchild while their son or daughter finishes middle school or high school. Then there is the rising epidemic of sexually transmitted diseases. Many of these diseases are incurable and many lead to pain, infertility and several are deadly. (I'm not just referring to AIDS.)

Whether you want your children to wait until marriage or to experiment freely with protected sex, unless you communicate openly with them how do you get your message across?

Research shows that one of the chief factors in determining a child's decisions on sex is how openly the parents communicated their views on sex. Communication doesn't mean the old standby one liner, "Don't have sex." It's about helping your children understand the ramifications of sex and making sure they are free to ask you questions to which they know they will get straight, truthful answers. It's about equipping them to make good decisions when you aren't there to guide them.

The goal of this book is to help you:

1. Become informed on the actual risks of sex.
2. Be prepared to openly communicate with your children the facts about sex.
3. Eliminate the embarrassment parents often feel when talking about sex with their children.
4. Equip your children to make good decisions about sex when you are not there to help them.

1

Your children are going to make decisions about sex. If you have taught them the "facts," they can make informed decisions. If not, then their decisions will be based on the information they get from friends, television, movies, and what they happen to feel when they find themselves in the heat of passion.

We've all heard of parents who have said, "If you get a girl pregnant" or "If you get pregnant, I'll kill you." I doubt many of these parents really meant what they said. They were just using a harsh method of communication in an effort to protect their children. In reality most of these parents would probably do what you or I would do if our children faced such a situation. We would cry with them, love them, hug them, and help them through the problems. After all, they are our children and we love them.

Although using such words as "I'll kill you" is harsh, it does show that parents intuitively want to help their children avoid pain and suffering. They just don't know how to communicate it. This book will provide you with current facts about sex and creative methods to communicate effectively with your children.

Best wishes as you
Empower Your Child to Succeed!

BOOK ONE

SECTION ONE

ABOUT THIS BOOK

Chapter 1

Why You Should be Talking
to Your Children about Sex

Kids are Searching for Answers

While speaking at an all-girls seminar in Houston, I asked how many of the young ladies were able to talk openly to their parents about sex. Out of about one hundred girls, only one raised her hand. Several others quickly responded, "I could never talk to my parents about sex!" They could, however, ask a total stranger nonstop questions on this subject. These girls, mostly ninth and tenth graders, asked questions like, "What is a wet dream?" "Is masturbation bad?" "What if my periods are not regular, is that okay?" "Why are guys so consumed with a girl's breasts?" "If a condom is used correctly every time you have sex, will it prevent sexually transmitted diseases?" "Can you get sexually transmitted diseases from oral sex?" "Can a girl get pregnant if the guy pulls out before he ejaculates?" These young ladies wanted answers. And they were going to get them anywhere EXCEPT from their parents.

There is nothing unusual about today's young people. They are just as curious about sex as you and I were when we were young. However, it's more important than ever before that they have good information so their decisions are based on facts and not on how they feel in the heat of passion.

If You're Not Talking, Who Is?

It's a fact. Your children are going to learn about sex. The question is – who is going to teach them?

Most children learn more about sex from television, magazines, books, and their friends than from their own parents. A great deal of what they learn is misleading. How often do you see a girl get pregnant on TV? It seldom happens. But in real life, one in five sexually active teenage girls get pregnant each year.[1] How often do people get sexually transmitted diseases (STDs) on TV or in the movies? Probably never. But in real life, one in four sexually active teens gets an STD every year.[2]

While parents may find it difficult to talk openly about this sensitive subject, discomfort does not alleviate the critical need to address it.

Parents Make a Difference

Studies are indicating that young people who are raised in homes where sex is openly discussed are much more likely to follow the advice of their parents regarding sexual activity. An article in *Time* magazine recently stated: "Recent studies indicate that many teens think parents are the most accurate source of information and would like to talk to them more about sex and sexual ethics but can't get their attention long enough . . . Parents haven't set boundaries, but they are expecting them."[3]

Taking a Strong Stand

It will be difficult to talk about sex with your children if you are not sure where you stand on this issue. The Sexual Revolution of the '60s promoted a lifestyle of free sex with multiple sexual partners. Through the years this behavior has sifted down to 12 and 13-year-olds. While most parents agree that young children should not be having sex, they are confused about when approval should be given. In the midst of their confusion many parents find it easier to turn their heads and remain silent on this sensitive subject and just hope everything will turn out okay.

But if parents really knew the dangers their children were facing today, they wouldn't be silent. Things have changed drastically since the '60s and '70s. The fact is your children are growing up in a time when sexual activity is now a matter of life and death, and I'm not just referring to AIDS.

For example, did you know the Human Papilloma Virus (HPV) is the most common sexually transmitted disease in America?[4] To make matters worse, this *incurable* disease is resulting in the death of thousands of women each year. The clincher is that condoms provide little to no protection.[5]

This book will bring you up to date on the current STD epidemic. It will also provide factual information about contraceptives so you can draw your own conclusions and decide where you stand. Once you have formed your own opinion, you will be able to confidently teach your child what is right and what is wrong based on your personal beliefs.

Getting Comfortable with Your Own Sexuality

Many parents avoid the subject of sex because they are not comfortable with their own sexuality. Many adults grew up with the impression that sex was dirty. Women have told me about their vivid memories of their mothers shaking their fingers in their faces and sternly exclaiming, "Sex is *very, very* bad and should be saved for your wedding night." Now *that* would give a girl something exciting to look forward to. Interestingly enough, many of the ladies said that statement kept them from having sex before marriage, but there is a good chance it also resulted in unhealthy attitudes about sex after marriage.

If you are uncomfortable with your sexuality, this book may provide helpful insights so you can gain a healthy perspective of sex. Sexual desires are normal and natural. Sexual relationships can result in fun and pleasure. But these same desires and relationships can be extremely destructive when misused or abused. One of the best things you can do for your children is to acquire your own healthy perspective of sex. Your positive attitude will rub off on your children.

Your Child Needs a Role Model

Whoever teaches your child about sex will likely become his or her primary role model in this area. That person will then play a major part in establishing your child's value system. If most of your child's sex education is coming from television and movies, then Hollywood becomes the primary role model. If it is the health teacher at school providing the education, then it's that teacher taking on this responsibility. Do you really want Hollywood or a total stranger from school playing such a major role in molding your child's value system?

Our children need positive role models, and this includes examples of healthy, long-term sexual relationships. The only image most teens have of sex today is hot, passionate sex on television and in the movies where everyone seems to jump from bed to bed. Most teens would be amazed to learn that a national study found that married people have more fulfilling sex lives than single people.[6] (This will be discussed in more detail later in the book.)

As a parent, you are a role model. It doesn't matter if you are married or a single parent. The question you need to ask yourself is this: Are you a positive or negative role model?

If you are married, it is good to let your children see hints of passion in your relationship. Children who see their parents hold hands or share a gentle kiss and hug can be reminded that love and passion don't just take place in Hollywood.

If you are a single parent, you have a great opportunity to demonstrate the same standards you expect of your children. By setting high standards for yourself, you become a powerful role model for your children as well as their friends. And I assure you – they are watching!

Whether you are married or single, what you are saying or not saying about sex will have a profound impact on the outcome of your child's life. Get over your hang-ups, know where you stand, become a positive role model, and talk openly to your children about sex!

A family that can talk about sex
together can talk about anything!

References

[1] The Alan Guttmacher Institute, *Sex and the American Teenager,* New York, NY 1994; 41.

[2] Kaiser Family Foundation and American Social Health Association, *STDs in America: How Many Cases and At What Cost?* Menlo Park, CA, 1998; 10.

[3] Stodghill, Ron, "Where'd You Learn That?" *Time;* June 15, 1998; 52-59.

[4] Kaiser Family Foundation and American Social Health Association, *STDs in America: How Many Cases and At What Cost?* Menlo Park, CA, 1998;18.

[5] National Institutes of Health. *Cervical Cancer. NIH Consensus Development Statement,* Online, April 1-3, 1996; 43(1), 1-30.

[6] Michael, Robert T., et al., *Sex in America*, New York: Little, Brown and Co., 1994; 124.

Chapter 2

How to Use This Book

Success does not just happen.
It takes knowledge and determination to make
choices that lead to lifelong success.

As I look back on my life and discuss growing up with others, I am struck by a very important fact. As children (and even adults) we didn't make bad decisions about our lives because we wanted to experience the pain of failure or wanted to get into trouble. No, we generally made bad decisions because:

1. We didn't have enough knowledge about the subject at hand to understand the ramifications of our actions.

2. We were too embarrassed by our lack of knowledge to ask for help.

3. We didn't have a logical decision-making process to follow, so our decisions were based on emotions.

4. We had not established clear goals for our lives to compare to immediate situations.

Children come into this world completely devoid of knowledge. How can we expect them to make good choices until they have the necessary tools to do so? Often these tools are only acquired later in the adult years. But wouldn't it be great if we could enable our children to obtain these tools long before they become adults?

Think of this book as a toolbox. Inside are tools which will empower your children to succeed. As they become skilled in using the various tools, they will learn that success requires:

> Knowledge and understanding (Tool #1)
> Learning from those with experience (Tool #2)
> Determination to succeed (Tool #3)

The benefits you can expect as a result of your child skillfully using the tools provided in this series are:

1. Your child's knowledge and understanding will expand.
2. Your relationship with your child will strengthen.
3. Your communication with your child will grow deeper.
4. Your child will begin making INFORMED decisions.

Fitting this Book to Your Needs

Whether you have toddlers and you're trying to prepare for those tough questions on the horizon or you have a house full of teenagers and you're trying to survive the dating years, this book will provide a wealth of knowledge.

There are two ways you can use this book. First, you can read the book and then share the information with your children when their questions or various situations arise. The other way is in conjunction with the student book TEENS Sex AND CHOICES. As you look through the third section of this book, you will see that it is actually designed to be the parent manual for the student book TEENS Sex AND CHOICES. If this is how you plan to use the book, the rest of this chapter will provide helpful hints on how to take your children through this series.

Remember, even if you aren't taking your children through this series, you will gain new insights and valuable information throughout the entire book.

How to Use this book with *TEENS Sex AND CHOICES*

Consider this book a teacher's manual. From cover to cover you will find a variety of creative ideas, helpful hints on parenting, as well as thought provoking discussion questions.

Each of your children will need their own copy of TEENS Sex AND CHOICES. At the end of this chapter is information on how to order additional items should you need extra copies.

At the conclusion of each chapter your children will complete a short workbook section. This allows them to apply each chapter to their own personal life. Next comes the **Family Discussion Questions**. This is where you come into the picture. After your children have finished reading each chapter and completed the workbook assignment, your family can have fun talking about your various points of view. Discussion questions have been provided at the end of each chapter. Notice in *this edition* most of the chapters have **Additional Discussion** questions for parents who want to take their discussion deeper. These additional questions *do not* appear in your child's book. This allows you to take the discussion as deep as you desire. You will also notice that in *this edition* there are also special notes to parents before each chapter. This will help prepare you for the chapter and should make your discussion time more enjoyable.

Who will benefit from TEENS Sex AND CHOICES?

TEENS Sex AND CHOICES is recommended for students 6th grade through college. However, you know your children and their maturity level and can best determine when to begin empowering your children to make informed decisions. Keep in mind, however, that your children are growing up in a sex saturated society where 10 and 11-year-old girls are getting pregnant.

How to Use TEENS Sex AND CHOICES with Your Children

A Family Gathering – You can read a chapter or listen to a tape with your children. (TEENS Sex AND CHOICES is also available on audio tape or CD. See the end of this chapter for ordering information.) At the end of each chapter have your children complete their workbook assignment privately. Then you can reassemble for the Family Discussion.

Students Working Alone – You can have each participating family member complete each chapter and workbook assignment privately and then come together for the Family Discussion.

Time Schedule – The time schedule is critical. If you go too fast, valuable information may be overlooked. Perhaps more importantly, *if you drag this out too long, your children may lose interest.* Therefore, a 30-day plan is recommended.

There are 15 chapters in TEENS Sex AND CHOICES. It will take your children about 20 to 30 minutes to read a chapter and complete their Workbook assignment. Family Discussions will probably take another 20 to 30 minutes. Therefore, if you assign one chapter in the book and workbook for one day, you can have your discussion on the next day. That way you are taking 30 minutes a day for 30 days to help your children make *CHOICES* that lead to lifelong success. That's not asking a lot when you consider the benefits!

Sticking with Your Plan – If you begin working through this material as a family, make a commitment to finish it as a family. By setting a schedule and making it a priority you are sending a strong message to your children that this is important.

If necessary, make a rule that there are to be no telephone conversations and no television until the daily assignment is complete. You might also consider taking the phone off the hook during Family Discussions. Remember: This is only for 30 minutes a day for 30 days.

Share Your Values – As you weave your values into each discussion the success of this endeavor will be enhanced. A child who grows up in a home with strong values will have a deep sense of self-respect and respect for others. Parents who lovingly share important information with their children are equipping, encouraging, and reinforcing values. These values build strong, responsible character.

Who Should Be Doing the Talking?

It seems the responsibility of talking about sex usually falls on the shoulders of dear old Mom. I'm not sure why this tends to happen, but it does. It's wonderful that mothers across the country are getting over their hang-ups and talking to their children about this sensitive subject. Obviously, when moms talk about sex it can really help, but when a father joins in the discussions – Wow! What a difference it can make. Instead of getting only the female side, the children are now learning attitudes and viewpoints from both male and female. This doesn't mean mothers should refrain from talking. It simply means fathers should join in and do their share so the children are hearing from both parents.

In situations where either mom or dad are not around or are unable to be involved in the discussions, it is far better to get one side than no side at all. Perhaps there is a relative or close friend whom you trust to become a positive role model for your children. Although they can't replace a missing parent, they might be able to join some of your discussions to add insights from the opposite sex.

A Special Note to Dads

What a father says or doesn't say about sex to his children can have a profound impact on their sexuality and self-image. A father who lovingly takes the time and patience to go through this book with his children is building lifelong memories and establishing strong family values. These values could actually mean the difference between life and death for your children. It can also mean the difference between a successful, bright future or a miserable life of failure for your child. What a difference a little of your time and words of wisdom can make.

A father told me he explained to his 10-year-old son that a day would come when his attitude toward "yucky old girls" would change. The dad smiled and said, "You know in a couple of years when my son has raging hormones, he's going to think back to our conversation and realize his father is an absolute genius. And if I was right about this, then perhaps I'll have other words of wisdom worth listening to as well."

A lady told me that on her 13th birthday her father announced to the entire family that he was going to allow her to start dating when she was sixteen. However, the dad went on to explain that he was requesting the first date on the evening of her 16th birthday. The next two birthdays served as a reminder that he would be taking her out on her first date. The day finally came. The two of them dressed up and he took her to an elegant restaurant. Throughout dinner the father talked about how proud he was of his daughter and what a beautiful young lady she had become. He told her stories about the day she was born and her first day of school. He then told her that from this day forward she could begin going out with young men. "However," he said, "I expect all the young men to treat you with the dignity and respect that I am treating you with tonight." The lady said her father set a wonderful example that night which had a tremendous impact on the rest of her life.

Fathers, you have a far more profound impact on your children than you will ever imagine. Don't pass up the incredible opportunities you have to guide, protect, and direct them.

Getting Your Child Involved

Your child may be the type who will eagerly go through this series. On the other hand, if you experience some resistance from your child, you might consider using your creative powers to provide positive incentives. For example, you could let your children know if they complete TEENS Sex AND CHOICES, including the workbook sections and all the family discussion *within the allotted time*, they will be allowed to . . . (You fill in the blank.)

I had a number of families test this material for me. Because I was on a tight schedule for going to print, I told each young person that I would give them fifty dollars if they completed the series with their parents within one month. I didn't think about it at the time, but what I was actually doing was offering these young people a challenge and a prize. To fulfill the challenge, each young person had to determine a plan of action. Sacrifices had to be made along the way to fulfill the task. It also required discipline and determination to succeed. A successful lifestyle is no different. To succeed there must be a definite plan of action. Sacrifices will have to be made in the midst of building self-discipline and determination.

If you feel a monetary reward might be helpful, don't forget grandparents. They may be thrilled to put up the prize money. Of course, the reward doesn't have to be money. You might tell your child he or she can go to the prom or upcoming school event *IF* the series is completed in the allotted time. There is always camp, a ski trip, or the onset of dating to be considered as leverage.

Whether you use parental authority or creative powers to provide incentive to get your children into this series, what may start as drudgery will probably end in fun family communication. It did for all the families who tested the material. Besides, it will be impossible to go through this material without gaining a great deal of valuable information.

I received a note last week from a mother telling me about the positive impact TEENS Sex AND CHOICES had on her daughter. She said, "Several moms have asked about the book because their daughters have remarked on the change in my daughter's attitude toward boys. I'm purchasing a second copy because I'm not willing to give mine up."

What is Discussed

This material accurately covers a variety of topics about sex. Proper names are used for body parts and accurate medical information is provided. Medical consultants for this series included an obstetrician and gynecologist, infertility specialist, pediatrician, behavioral pediatrician, and a psychologist.

Through this series your child will learn about:

The good and bad sides to sex
Problems of multiple sexual partners
Male and female reproductive systems
Menstruation/ovulation/menopause
Ejaculation and nocturnal emission
Sexual intercourse and conception
Multiple births, miscarriages and
  abortion
Facts on fetal development
Sexually transmitted diseases
Pregnancy
Dangers of oral sex, anal sex, and
  mutual masturbation
Emotional scars

Sexual abuse, rape and date rape
Lack of self-control
The failure rate of contraceptives
The purpose of dating
How far is too far
Why alcohol, drugs and sexual
  abstinence don't work together
The problems of pornography
The importance of setting goals
Importance of accountability partners
What to do if you stumble
What to do if you've already had sex
What clothes say about who you are
Creative ways to commit to abstinence

Three Important Points

#1 A child who goes through this book alone will still gain valuable information which will be helpful in making decisions about sex. However, a great opportunity will be missed in opening communication through the family discussion time. This book has been designed as a tool, not a replacement for parents. The information in each chapter is important, but the Family Discussion time is where the additional learning and bonding takes place.

#2 During the discussion time you may find that younger children will usually go along with whatever Mom and Dad say. But older children may not always agree with their parents. That's okay! *Just don't overreact!* And don't use this time to set rules or to discipline. This is meant to be a time of communication. *Give your child the right to think for himself and to disagree.* Remember, if you push too hard, you may push your child into rebellion. If you simply share information, he may eventually come around to your way of thinking. Children are not stupid. If they know the facts they generally come to good logical decisions.

#3 As your family works through this material, consider yourself a teacher. A good teacher always studies and prepares before class. Make sure you go through the material in its entirety before sharing it with your children. Review the discussion questions prior to your family time together. Remember, you can allow the discussion to go as deep as you desire and add additional information as you see fit.

My best wishes to you as you help your child make
CHOICES that lead to lifelong success!

Additional Items Available in the
TEENS Sex AND CHOICES Series

ABC's of the Birds and Bees for Parents of Toddlers to Teens – This book is designed to prepare parents for tough issues regarding their children and sex. Included are 50 FAQ (Frequently Asked Questions). This book is also designed as a companion parent manual to *TEENS Sex AND CHOICES*

TEENS Sex AND CHOICES – This book will educate young and old alike on the issues of sex as it opens the doors of communication within the family. Each book also includes a workbook section and family discussion questions.

Audio Tapes and CD - The book, *TEENS Sex AND CHOICES*, is also available on audio tapes and CD. Mike Frazier reads the book with the exception of the fourth chapter, "I Had a Dream." In this chapter, the author tells her own personal story. (Note: Workbook questions and Family Discussion Questions are not included on the tapes or CD.)

Certificates – The student "Commitment Certificate" and the parent "Commitment of Love" certificates are suitable for framing and are great additions to this series. The certificates are inscribed as follows:

Student Commitment Certificate

I am going to strive to succeed at the lifestyle of sexual abstinence until marriage. From this day forward, I will strive to develop the self-control, self-respect, and self-discipline necessary to save myself for my spouse on my wedding day. I want to experience freedom from STDs, pregnancy, and emotional scars. I also want to experience freedom to fulfill my dreams and goals. This is not going to be an easy lifestyle, but I believe I can succeed. When I feel weak, I will ask for your help. If I stumble, I know I can tell you and you will still love me.

Parent Commitment of Love

I love you. As your parent I desire to see you succeed at the lifestyle of sexual abstinence until marriage. I want you to experience freedom from STDs, pregnancy, and emotional scars. I also want you to experience the freedom to succeed with your dreams and goals. I know this is not going to be an easy lifestyle, but I believe you have the ability to succeed! When you feel weak, I will be here to encourage you. If you fail, please allow me to help you. If I appear upset or angry, please forgive me. I am not angry at you but at the circumstances. My anger will pass, but my love for you will be forever.

See the Order Form in the back of
this book to order these items.

BOOK ONE

SECTION TWO

ANSWERS TO TOUGH QUESTIONS

Chapter 3

50 FAQs
(Frequently Asked Questions)

What Parents Want to Know About Sex and Their Children
From Toddlers to Teens

I answer the following questions with the assumption that you want your children to wait for sex until marriage. This approach has been taken because:

1. Encouraging your children to wait is the more difficult approach (i.e., it's always easier at the moment to give your children permission to do something than to ask them to deny themselves.)

2. Abstinence until marriage is the only GUARANTEED way to avoid STDs, pregnancy and the deep emotional pain which might result from sex before marriage.

This book has been designed to help your children learn the facts about sexual activity and to provide you the opportunity to interject your values. If you want your children to be sexually active before marriage, change the dialogues as appropriate.

1. When should we have "The Talk?"

I am personally opposed to the "Sex Talk." The reason is because most parents who have "The Talk" with their child tend to wait until they are 13 or 14. Then they nervously mumble a few things about sex, walk out of the room with sweating palms, a pounding heart and a deep satisfaction that they had fulfilled yet one more duty of responsible parenting.

While it may be true that one brief, clumsy talk may have had an impact back when you were growing up, believe me, it's not going to cut it today. Remember, sex is everywhere! Music, magazines, television, movies, the Internet, even commercials reek of S-E-X! And I assure you your child can't help but notice!

So if you were planning to wait until your child is 13 or 14 to say a few words you better think again, because you'll be too late! Teachers tell me children in first, second, and third grade are talking about sex. Now they may not have all their facts straight at this young age, but it doesn't stop them from talking and even experimenting.

It isn't a question of whether your child will learn about sex at an early age, it's a question of who will teach him – you or his friends? If you want your child to share your values about sex, you need to begin talking to him before the other children at school start filling his mind with distorted information. Then, when he does start hearing information at school, he will be able to discern fact from fiction as he gains a greater respect and appreciation for you.

Let's begin by considering two critical stages of your child's life and what you can do in these early years to begin opening communication on this subject.

Birth - Now you certainly aren't going to explain the facts of life to a newborn, but you can get started on the right foot by using proper names for body parts.

Why is it that when we are dealing with small children we call that thing we breathe with a nose, those things at the end of our hands fingers, and those things at the end of our feet toes? Then when it comes to the area between our legs we use such dumb names? Is it because we don't want to embarrass the baby? No. A baby wouldn't know to be embarrassed by words. Could it possibly be that we as adults are uncomfortable saying terms such as vagina and penis?

If a mother or father changed their baby boy's diaper and said, "Let's clean your penis," would the baby blush with embarrassment because the word penis was used instead of wee-wee or pee-pee? Of course not, the baby could care less what word is used. So, who will benefit from using the correct terms? That's right – the parents! If you can get over your hang-ups about using proper names while your child is an infant, you have cleared the first big hurdle in talking about sex.

Three to eight-years-old - Once again, you don't need to sit a three-year-old down and explain the facts of life, but if he is asking questions, you need to be prepared to give him answers. It isn't unusual for a three or four-year-old to ask, "Where do babies come from?" (This question will be addressed in #4.) This is often the result of a new baby brother or sister which might be on the way or a friend or relative who might be expecting a baby. Then again some children are just inquisitive and will naturally begin to ask these questions.

The most important thing you can do is be prepared to answer this question. In fact, you need to welcome such questions. If your children are not coming to you, they will be going to their friends. Your immediate response to this first question could open the door for a lifetime of heart-to-heart talks, or it could close the doors forever. (But hey – no pressure!)

2. How do I answer those early questions?

There are four important rules to remember when talking to young children about sex:

1. Understand what your child wants to know
2. Use real terms
3. Be honest
4. Keep your answers short

When you hear that question, "Where do babies come from?" it will, no doubt, be when you least expect it and will catch you totally off guard. So here's a suggestion to help you quickly recover from the initial shock of this unexpected question. Quickly turn to your child, SMILE, and say, "Wow! What a great question. What made you think of that?"

By doing this, you are doing three things. First you are stalling – trying to collect your thoughts and remembering how you were going to answer this question. Second you are praising your child for coming to you with his or her questions and thus inviting future questions. Last you are finding out what triggered the question and what it is your child really wants to know.

So, when you said, "Wow! What a great question. What made you think of that?" Your child may quickly respond, "Well, Jennifer said she was from Chicago and I was just wondering where I was from."

Now you know exactly how to answer. Wasn't that easy!

3. What if the questions come in the middle of a crowded area?

These early questions often come at the most inopportune times like at the check out stand at the grocery story or at a family gathering. Should this happen it is important that you not laugh at your child or make him feel uncomfortable for asking such questions. Instead, praise him for asking such an intelligent question and let him know you will answer his question as soon as you get home where it isn't so noisy and busy. Then make sure you do just that. If your child has asked once, it is on his mind. Don't avoid the situation. Welcome it as a teachable moment.

4. How do I explain where babies come from to a young child?

If your child really wants to know where she came from, you need to be prepared to approach the subject. Remember, you don't need to tell her all the facts of life at once. Rather offer her the information she seems to be searching for. Perhaps the following simple statement might help.

"Mommies have a special place called a uterus, and that is where babies grow. It's about right here," the mother says as she points to her lower abdomen. "A uterus is sort of like a balloon that stretches as the baby grows. Remember when we saw Mrs. Jones at the grocery store yesterday and how big her stomach looked? Well, that is because she has a little baby growing inside her uterus."

The child might be satisfied at this point and run off to play. The mother feels good because she knows she has taken the first small step in teaching her child about sexual reproduction. She also knows she has just taken a giant leap in opening the doors to a lifetime of communication.

It is very possible the child will come right back and ask the very same question a few days or several months later. You should be prepared to give a repeat performance knowing your child is simply trying to understand this new concept. As new questions surface in the child's mind, she will automatically go to you because **you made her feel comfortable and welcomed her questions.**

5. How do I explain how the baby gets out?

The next obvious question you can expect is, "How does the baby get out?"
When asked, apply the same four rules:

1. Understand what your child wants to know
2. Use real terms
3. Be honest
4. Keep your answer short

"What a great question! I'm so proud that you think of such good questions. Mommies have a special opening between their legs called a vagina. When the time is right, the baby comes out of the vagina and then the mommy and daddy get to hold and cuddle their little baby."

6. How does the baby get inside the mommy?

At some point the inevitable question will be asked: "How does the baby get inside the Mommy?"

Get down on your child's level with creative information that he can understand. There are some great picture books at the bookstore or library that might make this a little easier. There are also a variety of illustrations that could be used. One such example would be as follows:

27

"Daddy, how does the baby get inside the mommy?" the child asks inquisitively.

"What a great question. I'm proud of you for asking me about this. First of all it takes a man and a woman to have a baby," the father replies. "And it's sort of like planting flowers. Do you remember when we wanted flowers in the back yard a few months ago? What did we do?"

"We made holes in the ground," the child quickly responds.

"That's right. And what else did we do?" the father asks.

"We dropped seeds in the holes and covered them up. Then you put fertilizer on them and I watered them. And then we got flowers," the child enthusiastically replies.

"Exactly! You have a great memory! So when a mommy and daddy want a baby they first have to have a special place for the baby to grow, just like the flowers. Do you remember what that special place inside a lady is called where the baby grows?"

"A ut-er something," the child answers remembering a previous discussion.

"That's right, a uterus. You learn fast! Actually, women already have seeds inside them. They don't feel them, but they are there. Now if we took one seed from the package of flower seeds and put it on the table it wouldn't grow because it has to have dirt, water, and fertilizer. Well, the seeds inside a woman can't grow either until they receive something kind of like fertilizer. Now who do you suppose gets to fertilize the egg?"

"The daddy?" the child asks curiously.

"That's right! Daddies get the joy of putting the fertilizer inside the mommy. Actually, it is called sperm. And the sperm fertilizes the egg."

"But how does the daddy get the sperm inside the mommy?"

"He uses his penis. Gently and lovingly he places it inside the mommy's vagina which is a special place between a mommy's legs. The sperm comes out of the daddy and goes inside the mommy. This is called having sex or sexual intercourse. Some people call it making love because this is a special way a husband and wife give love to each other. This is very good and husbands and wives like to do this. In fact, it is so good and so special that we *do not* do this with anyone else but each other. We also only do it when we are all alone because it is a very private time for us. And someday, after you get married you will be able to have sexual intercourse and make love to your wife. And it will be so special and so beautiful for the two of you."

"I think it all sounds kind of yucky!" the child replies.

"Well it probably does right now, but when you get older it will begin to sound pretty good. You know when you were a baby you were born with an appetite. Do you know what you were hungry for?"

"Milk?" the child quickly replies.

"Exactly!" says the father. "You just loved your bottle of milk. But what would have happened if I had given you some fried chicken and corn on the cob when you were a little baby?"

"I would have choked."

"That's right," responds the father. "It could have been very dangerous! Because you weren't ready for that kind of food, and you didn't have an appetite for it either. But in time you gained an appetite for fried chicken and corn on the cob, didn't you? And now you love it and eat it every chance you get.

"Well, that's sort of how it is with sex. You don't have an appetite for sex yet, but you will! When you get older, sex will begin to sound pretty good.   Sort of like fried chicken. But remember, sex is *so* good that you will want to save it and do it only with the special person you marry. So, although sex may not sound too good now, someday when you have an appetite for it, you will look forward to it and it will be very good!"

Now, was that embarrassing? I certainly hope not! The parents' attitude makes all the difference in the world. Sharing this information in a light-hearted, loving attitude will help the child think of sex as something good . . . and it is!

7. What if my child never asks questions?

Even if your children are not asking you questions, they will be hearing about sex from their friends at school beginning at a young age. Therefore, if they are not asking questions by the time they are in the first or second grade, it may be necessary to help open the doors of communication.

Try having the following discussion with your first or second grader:

> Honey, I know at school you may have heard some kids talk about sex. If you haven't, you probably will soon. I want you to know you can come to me and ask me any questions you have about sex. But for right now I want you to know that sex is something that is very good. It is something that husbands and wives do in the privacy of their bedroom to show each other how much they love each other. And anytime you want to talk about this we will.

You might also try this – the next time you see a pregnant lady, nudge your child and say, "Hey, see that pregnant lady? I remember when you were inside me. I just loved feeling you kick." (Or Dad can say, "I remember when you were inside your Mom. We had so much fun feeling you kick.")

Neither of these discussions are embarrassing. But you used real terms – sex and pregnant. And you casually let your child know that it's okay to have this type of discussion.

If your child still isn't asking questions by the third grade, I would recommend you go ahead and explain sex in a simple way. If you don't, your child will be learning from friends instead of you. Make sure you use the same rules:

1. Use real terms
2. Be honest
3. Keep your discussion short

If you feel uncomfortable or nervous, admit that to your child. The first time I talked with my daughters I was really nervous. I started the discussion by just saying, "No one ever talked to me about sex. And it feels kind of weird to talk about this, but I want to be the one to explain it to you. So if I sound a little uncomfortable or nervous, would you just be patient with me? I promise I'll get better as we go along." Both my daughters patted me on the arm sympathetically and said, "Sure Mom, we'll be patient." That really helped ease the tension for all of us!

Another helpful suggestion is that you share the information while you're on a walk or sitting on a porch. In either case, you aren't looking eye to eye but just looking out in the distance as you talk.

You can start the discussion off the same way as before.

> Honey, I know kids at school are probably talking about sex. If you haven't heard about it yet, you will soon. I want to be the one who gives you the information because a lot of kids have some weird ideas about sex. Sex is something that husbands and wives do to show each other how much they love each other. They usually do this in the privacy of their bedroom, because it is a special and private expression of love between the two of them. When a couple has sex or makes love they start by kissing and hugging. Then the husband places his penis inside his wife's vagina (a special opening between her legs.) They both enjoy this because it feels good. A special fluid called sperm comes out of the husband's penis into the wife's vagina. If his sperm reaches one of her eggs, a baby may be made. Isn't that incredible!
>
> I know that right now this sounds strange. It did when I first heard about sex. But when you are a teenager, you will begin having sexual desires and thoughts. That is normal and natural. But it is important that you learn to control those sexual desires and save yourself for the person you marry. I promise that someday when you are older you will look forward to making love with your wife (or husband). Now remember, anytime you want to talk about this we will.

I have had more parents tell me they were amazed how well their children responded when they had this type of discussion. Sharing this information is usually easier with younger children than it is with teenagers. Remember that your six-year-old still has you high on a pedestal and believes your every word.

I hate to be the one to break the news, but it is inevitable that you will fall from the pedestal when your child becomes a teenager. This will occur at about the same time he or she begins to question your every word. That doesn't mean that if you have never talked to your teenager about sex that you shouldn't try. It simply means you have to work a little harder.

8. Can I give my child too much information?

I have found that most psychologists believe parents have a tendency to err on the side of not telling their children enough information. These same psychologists seem to agree our children will take in the amount of information they are capable of receiving. If we tell them too much, it will merely go over their heads.

It might be helpful to practice these conversations with your spouse or a friend. Even practicing this dialogue in front of a mirror can be very helpful in preparing such a talk. Try to be relaxed and carry on this discussion casually.

Remember, by the time your children reach the second or third grade, they will learn about sex from their friends. However, the method and terms will no doubt be crude, filled with inaccuracies, and perhaps terrifying to them unless they have been educated properly at home by loving parents.

9. What if my child talks about his penis in public?

Once a child knows he has a penis, or she has a vagina, many parents live in fear that their child will use this term in public. Would you be concerned if your child talked about his elbow or knee in public? No, because as adults we are comfortable with these terms. Once again the problem is not with the child using a correct term. The problem is that we as adults are not comfortable with the words penis and vagina.

To ease your concern, it would certainly be appropriate to explain to your child that it would be better if he did not talk about his penis (or her vagina) in public. You can simply explain that his penis is located in a private area of his body. That is why people wear clothes over this area. That is also why we close the bathroom door when we go to the bathroom. Since this is a private matter, we don't talk about it in public settings.

This would also be a good time to explain that no one has the right to touch your child in this "private" area. Sexual abuse will be discussed in question #27 as well as Chapter 10 in TEENS Sex AND CHOICES.

10. What if my young child masturbates?

Masturbating or playing with one's genitals is common for small children. It often becomes a habit similar to stuttering, sucking a thumb, or intense rocking. Children often do this because they are bored, tired, or stressed. A new sibling, a move to a new house, an intense TV show, or too much TV, might bring it on. If you make a big deal about it or punish your child, you may only make matters worse.

Try to break this habit with the following solutions. If your child is watching an intense TV show, turn off the TV and ask him to play a game with you. If your child is bored, hand him a toy or ask him to help you make some cookies. If your child is under too much stress because of potty training, rigid rules at dinner, or parents who are arguing, lighten up. Hugging and cuddling your child might reassure her and lessen the problem. You might also want to make sure your child is not wearing underwear and clothes that are too tight.

If the problem continues you might want to consult your physician, because this could be a sign of a physical or medical problem such as pinworms, depression, or sexual abuse.

11. What if I catch my child playing doctor with a friend?

First and foremost, DO NOT overreact. Overreacting may build walls that may never come down. Remember that children are curious by nature. So stay calm and look at this as a teachable moment.

With a calm voice simply tell the children that sexual activity is a private matter between husbands and wives, not friends. Then suggest they get dressed and come into the kitchen and offer to work a puzzle with them, or play a game, or make some cookies. By getting involved in an activity with them you are reinforcing the fact that you are not upset.

Make sure you tell the parents of the other child what happened and how you handled the situation.

12. What does character have to do with sex?

Sex education is not just about sexual intercourse. Sex, love, and character are closely intertwined. Preschool and grade school years are critical when it comes to teaching your child right from wrong. The child you carefully nurture today may be the teenager who is capable of saying no to drugs, alcohol, smoking and sex tomorrow. Remember, good character doesn't just happen. It must be taught with diligence and patience.

Unless you teach your child not to lie, he will not know it is wrong. How will he ever know it is wrong to cheat on a test or steal unless you take the time to teach him these values?

Find creative ways to instill values. For example, while helping your child study for a spelling test or math exam you could say, "I am so proud that you study so hard for your grades. You know when I was young, some of the kids cheated on tests because they were too lazy to study. I'm glad our family doesn't cheat and that honesty is important to us."

The best way you can instill values into your child is to model strong character. If you are respectful of others, he will come to know and understand the importance of showing respect. Not only will he tend to be more respectful of others he will also have a higher regard and respect for you. (What goes around comes around.) If you tell the truth, your child will come to understand honesty and being truthful.

Last week I was talking to a 25-year-old newlywed. After telling me he was a virgin on his wedding night, I asked him what was the primary factor that kept him living the abstinent lifestyle before marriage. Without giving it a second thought, he responded, "My Dad." He went on to explain, "You see, all the years I was growing up he modeled respect by the way he treated friends, family and business associates. He taught me from the time I could talk to say, 'Yes, sir' and 'No, sir.' I determined it was impossible to show my dates respect and ask them to have sex. Respect and premarital sex just don't go hand in hand."

A college student shared with me how her mother taught her about honesty. But in this case the mother explained that honesty was not always the best policy. She explained to her daughter that telling small lies, also known as a white lie, was not wrong. If it kept people from having their feelings hurt or made a situation better for everyone concerned, then it was okay. This character trait of telling white lies came full circle when the little girl grew up. She said that in high school she got very good at telling her mother "little white lies." She said she didn't give it a second thought. After all, it was her mother who taught her how to do it. With just a few "white lies" here and there her mother stayed off her back, she got to do what she wanted, and everyone was happy. Of course, she went on to tell me she got pregnant when she was 16 and got herpes in college. Whether you know it or not, you are modeling character traits for your children. The question is – are they positive or negative traits?

Controlling one's sexual appetite requires strong character. Not only is it important to respect yourself, you must hold those you date in high regard. Self-control is important even though controlling raging hormones is extremely difficult! Honesty is also important as you boldly explain where you stand on the subject of sex – even if others might laugh. Determination to succeed, faithfulness, discipline – all of these are critical for those who are striving for sexual abstinence.

It comes as no surprise that teenagers who successfully live the abstinent lifestyle are also less likely to be involved in drugs, alcohol and smoking. This is discussed further in Chapter 11 of TEENS Sex AND CHOICES.

13. Who should do the talking – Mom or Dad?

When it comes to the first talk, the best answer I have is either or both. If one parent is more comfortable with this subject than the other, then that parent should be the designated spokesperson.

After the initial talk, all you are doing is having on-going dialogues as you make the most of every opportunity that comes along. In other words, most of your conversations will not be planned. They just happen as you are driving home from the big game, while you're watching a TV show, after seeing a billboard along the highway, or when you're telling your child good night. How great if both Mom and Dad are willing participants.

If you are a single parent or if your spouse is not working with you in this, there is absolutely nothing wrong with you rolling up your sleeves and taking this project on all alone! You might want to find a friend or relative of the opposite sex to talk with your children occasionally so they can gain both the male and female perspective. Just make sure this person holds your same values.

14. I'm nervous about talking to my child. Won't it be obvious?

Yes. It probably will be, but maybe not as obvious as you might think. The best solution is just to admit you are uncomfortable and tell your child you hope to get better. And then practice, practice, practice! Remember, the more you talk the easier it will get.

One of the main reasons I wrote TEENS Sex AND CHOICES is for this very purpose. I know most parents want their children to have good information about sex. But I also know most parents find it difficult to talk about this sensitive subject. Therefore, the book will do the difficult part of telling your child all the information he or she needs to know, and all you have to do is take part in the Family Discussion Questions. I worked hard to keep the discussions fun and comfortable.

15. What if my teenager doesn't want to talk about sex?

Many parents tell me they have tried talking to their children about sex, but their child shows no interest. Or perhaps you have gotten this kind of response from your child, "Oh Mom, you don't have to worry about me, I'm not interested in sex."

Let me make one comment and a suggestion that might help. First the comment: If we were discussing dental hygiene and your child had this same uninterested attitude you would *not* say to your child, "Okay dear, we will discuss this subject in a year or two when you seem a little more interested."

No. Undoubtedly, you would sit your child down and have a discussion about caring for his teeth – whether he wanted it or not.

Now, isn't your child's physical and emotional well being at least as important as his teeth?

Perhaps there are ways you could approach the subject that might be more inviting to your child. A heavy, serious format may automatically make your child feel uncomfortable. Try to be creative and upbeat in your discussion.

Recently, a lady told me she had heard me speak at an adult seminar. She said the mere thought of talking to her two daughters about sex terrified her. She had actually worked hard to avoid this subject for years, and her daughters never showed any desire to have a discussion. However, she went home that evening determined that sex had to become an open subject in their home.

That night she walked into her daughters' bedroom and simply said, "Tonight, I heard a lady talk about how she got pregnant when she was 17. It made me start thinking. What options does a girl have if she finds out she is pregnant?" She listened as her daughters began talking about marriage, single parenting, adoption and abortion. They discussed the problems of each option, which led to a discussion of which option they would choose and how that would affect their dreams and goals. She said for two hours she and her daughters talked, laughed, giggled and shared from their hearts.

A couple of nights later she went in their room again. This time she said, "You know girls, the other night I also learned about some diseases. I have never even heard about most of these. Have you ever heard of Chlamydia?"

Again, a couple of hours went by and the three of them discussed this intimate subject without being embarrassed or uncomfortable. The mother proudly smiled as she said to me, "I can talk to my children about sex now! And the best part is, they know they can ask me anything they want."

Creative ways to stimulate conversation – If your child doesn't seem interested in talking about sex, try a different approach. The following ideas might help.

- Tell a friend, either in person or on the phone, about some of the sexually transmitted diseases. Just make sure your child is in earshot and can overhear the discussion. Eventually, your child may be willing to join in the conversation.

- When you see a pregnant woman, talk about what it was like when you were pregnant. Describe the joy, excitement and pain of pregnancy and childbirth.

- If you have a friend or relative who is pregnant, ask if you and your child could place your hands on her abdomen and feel the baby move.

- Get some pets such as gerbils, dogs, or cats and let them have babies. This would allow your child to understand reproduction, gestation, periods, and the birth process. This can be exciting and educational for children of all ages. Make sure you are willing to take on the responsibility of caring for these animals and their offspring before you try this.

- Check books out of the library which discuss reproduction of animals. You and your child can find out which living creatures give live births and which ones lay eggs. What animals have one mate for life? Which creatures kill their mates after mating? What is the gestation period for different animals? What responsibility does the male have in various species? How do various creatures feed their young? This can be fascinating, educational and lots of fun for young and old alike! Makes for great dinner conversation as well!

- Many of the educational television stations have wonderful programs on reproduction, fetal development and birth of animals and insects. These are interesting and can encourage on-going discussions.

- Are you a hunter? A father once told me he and his son spent a day hunting rabbits. At the end of the day they skinned the rabbits, and then the father used this opportunity to describe the male and female reproduction systems to his son. Instead of being embarrassed the son was fascinated.

16. My child and I aren't communicating well. What can I do?

As children get older, the methods of communicating with them must change. As we all know, children reach the age when they begin to think for themselves, and they no longer ask "how high" when the parents say "jump." Your family may have been sailing along so well, your kids doing whatever you ask, and then one day they suddenly begin to balk. This isn't necessarily rebellion. It may simply be a natural part of growing up.

As a child begins to question his mom and dad, the parents must learn to communicate patiently with logical reasons and explanations. If parents don't patiently work with their children during this changing time, rebellion may indeed quickly follow.

17. My teenager and I are always arguing. What should I do?

To help reduce arguments, pick your battles carefully. Constant complaining about petty issues will only harden your child and cause a lack of respect for you. If, however, your child wants to do something that is wrong, don't argue. Simply say no and explain why this is not acceptable and then end the discussion. If your child does it anyway, you need to determine a suitable punishment so your child learns that bad choices have bad consequences. It would be better for your child to learn this from you than from serious consequences outside the home later.

Next time you start to argue, ask yourself the following question: Is it wrong for my child to ———————— (fill in the blank with what you are arguing about) or do I just not like it.

For example, if you find out your teenage son or daughter has been drinking, don't argue about the situation. Drinking for a minor is always wrong. Therefore, instead of arguing, establish a suitable punishment and then make sure you carry it out. Let your child know the consequences will be much tougher if this happens again. The punishment should be tough enough that your child will not want to go through this again.

Now if you just don't like the new shade of purple your daughter has chosen for her fingernails, don't waste your time or energy arguing. There are a lot worse things she could do than wear purple fingernail polish. If her school allows it, maybe you should tolerate it as well. Save your complaining for more serious situations. Besides, it's possible she's selected purple just to rile you. If you don't react, the problem may resolve itself.

18. Is it necessary to talk to my son or just my daughter?

It is just as important to talk to your son as your daughter. While it is true that girls are more susceptible to STDs than boys, young men need to understand the lifelong complications of certain STDs such as herpes, HPV, and AIDS. Boys also need to know about DNA testing and child support. All these issues will be discussed in detail in TEENS Sex AND CHOICES.

There is also a reversed situation occurring today. While many young men are now making a commitment to sexual abstinence until marriage, there are girls considering these guys as a challenge. "Watch me," a girl will proudly boast. "I'll be the one to bring him down."

Yes, you need to work with your sons as well as your daughters.

19. When is it okay for sexual activity to begin?

There are many groups encouraging teens not to have sex until they are sure they are ready. But I assure you, two 14 year-olds in the heat of passion will quickly determine, "We're ready!" But what are they ready for? Sex? Evidently so. A lifelong commitment? I doubt it. A baby? Probably not. AIDS, cancer, sterility? No way! Just because the hormones are telling them they are ready for sex does not mean they are ready for all that goes along with their actions.

But what about high school students, college-aged students or single adults? What is the magic age when it becomes *okay* to start having sex? Many would say when a person is mature enough to practice safe sex. Others would say condoms, pills and injections only reduce the chances of pregnancy, AIDS, cancer, and sterility. They

40

would prefer to go with guaranteed protection of abstinence until marriage.

It is important that you know where you stand on this subject before working with your children. You need to determine if it is wrong to have sex before marriage and if contraceptives will provide enough protection for your child. TEENS Sex AND CHOICES will give you information to help you think through these issues.

20. Isn't waiting until marriage a religious issue?

While it is true that nearly all major religions hold strong convictions that sex outside marriage is wrong, the concept of abstinence until marriage goes beyond religion. Today, sexual abstinence is a health issue. You will learn about the STD epidemic in Chapters 6, 7, and 8 of TEENS Sex AND CHOICES.

If you are coming from a religious background, I recommend you carefully study what your religion says about sex before marriage and understand why you hold these beliefs. This can be helpful to both you and your child in your family discussions.

21. Would it be better to live together before marriage?

Many studies indicate just the opposite. Sociologists at the University of Wisconsin stated that, "Recent national studies in Canada, Sweden and the U.S. found that cohabitation increased rather than decreased the risk of marital dissolution." They also found that "cohabitation is associated with greater marital conflict and poorer communication."[1]

Another study documented in the *Journal of Marriage and the Family* stated that the divorce rate is 50 percent higher among those who lived together before marriage.[2]

An Australian study found that couples who cohabited before marriage were more likely to divorce than those who did not cohabit before marriage. They found that couples who lived together before marriage also "separated more often, sought counseling more often and regarded marriage as a less important part of their lives than those who did not live together before marriage."[3]

22. Should I put my teenage daughter on the pill?

Many parents feel they are being responsible by putting their 8th or 9th grade daughter on birth control pills. While these parents mean well, they need to realize they are actually giving their daughter permission to have sex. I've had girls tell me they weren't even thinking about having sex until their mothers put them on the pill. Once they were on the pill, there was nothing to prevent them from having sex.

Another important consideration is that the pill does not prevent STDs. This issue is discussed further in the Note to Parents in Chapter 12, "The Search for Perfect Protection" in TEENS Sex AND CHOICES.

A recent study published in the *Journal of the American Medical Association* stated that sexual activity among teenagers goes down when parents tell their children they disapprove of them having sex and disapprove of them using contraceptives. In other words, by simply saying, "I don't want you to have sex" and NOT providing contraceptives, your child is more likely not to have sex.[4]

Actually, the best protection from pregnancy and STDs does not come in the form of pills, injections, or implants. The best protection you can offer your child is your time. Studies are showing that pregnancy rates are lower among teenagers who have a greater number of shared activities with their parents. Go places, do things, and find hobbies to share with your children.[5]

23. My child is already having sex. What should I do?

That's a tough question and one I think you should carefully consider. Many people would encourage you to get your child on some form of contraceptives. Chapter 12 of TEENS Sex AND CHOICES will provide you with information about the leading forms of contraceptives, including their failure rates. While it seems logical that some form of protection is better than no protection, you also need to realize that by providing contraceptives you will be giving your child permission to have sex.

Young people are often left confused when Mom or Dad says, "I don't want you to have sex, but if you do, make sure you use a condom." Parents need to know where they stand on this subject and give a straight answer. Do you care if your child has sex or not? Yes or no. This is a tough issue and the question is discussed in more detail in the Note to Parents in Chapter 12 "The Search for Perfect Protection" of TEENS Sex AND CHOICES.

Just because your child has become sexually active does not mean he or she will continue in this lifestyle. Many young people who have had sex are now making a commitment to abstinence. Your guidance and direction could help your child to do the same.

According to the Centers for Disease Control and Prevention (CDC), approximately 25 percent of the teens who have had sex are now committed to abstinence.[6] I am president and founder of Aim for Success, Inc. We are one of the largest providers of abstinence programs in the nation. At the conclusion of our programs we offer an anonymous, voluntary survey. We have now surveyed over a quarter of a million students and come up with the same number as the CDC – 25 percent of the sexually active students have made a commitment to abstinence.

Making a commitment to sexual abstinence is not easy. Making a commitment after experiencing sex is even harder – but not impossible! The best thing you can offer your child is love, understanding, and good information. How can your child make good choices about sex without good information?

If you and your child go through *TEENS Sex AND CHOICES,* your child will gain the necessary knowledge and understanding to make an informed decision. Your child will learn that it is never too late to begin making good choices. While he cannot undo the past, he can prevent future risks.

Just remember that while you can require your child to go through TEENS Sex AND CHOICES with you, you cannot force him or her to accept your way of thinking. The harder you push, the greater chance of rebellion. Going through the material with the attitude that this is merely a way to obtain good, updated information may help your child's acceptance. It may also help that I never say in the book, "Don't have sex!" I let the facts speak for themselves – and they speak very loudly!

Having a sexually active child often puts a great strain on the family relationship. You must realize you are not responsible for your child's decisions. You are, however, responsible for providing good information. Once you provide the information and state your values, your child must make his or her own decisions. If your child continues with the sexual activity, I encourage you to diligently work to love your child unconditionally. That doesn't mean you open your home for your child's sexual encounters or that you condone what he or she is doing. It simply means you keep demonstrating love despite the rebellion against your values. Then, when the consequences come (and they probably will) you need to keep providing love. This doesn't mean you fix the problems (you can't fix an incurable STD or emotional scars), but you can gently remind your child that it is never too late to begin making good choices.

The TEENS Sex AND CHOICES series also provides certificates for students and parents. You might want to consider the Parent Commitment of Love certificate. It is described at the conclusion of Chapter Two under Additional Available Items.

24. Is it wrong for teenagers to masturbate?

There is nothing wrong with a teenager wanting to know how his or her body works. And it would be best not to make a big deal about it. In chapter 15 of TEENS Sex AND CHOICES, I explain to teenagers, however, that if they want to be successful at sexual abstinence until marriage their goal should be to gain control of their bodies and minds. Masturbating requires a person to concentrate on sexual fantasies instead of controlling their thoughts.

In addition, a person who masturbates on a regular basis will probably NOT be satisfied with self-gratification for very long. Mutual masturbation, oral, anal or vaginal sex would be the logical next steps. If those partners have had any type of sexual contact with someone else, there could be a problem with STDs.

25. Is oral sex safe?

No. Sexually transmitted diseases can be spread through oral sex. In fact, sores from herpes, syphilis, HPV, etc. can develop around the mouth and throat area as a result of oral sex.

Parents need to realize that oral sex is becoming the sex of choice among 7th and 8th grade students. Teenagers feel safe with oral sex because they know there won't be a pregnancy and they can still call themselves virgins. Unfortunately, most of them do not know about the risk of STDs. Chapter Six in TEENS Sex AND CHOICES explains the dangers of oral sex.

26. What is outer course?

Outer course is a slang term that refers to doing everything but "going all the way." Similar terms are mutual masturbation and dry sex. (Although there is nothing dry about dry sex.) This would include touching under clothes, removing clothes, bathing or taking a shower together.

Some groups promote these methods as healthy and safe for teenagers since a pregnancy would be extremely rare using these methods. The problem is, however, that STDs can still be transmitted when two bodies come into skin to skin contact. And as far as preventing a pregnancy, how long do you think two teenagers will be content putting their naked bodies together without going all the way?

Outer course, mutual masturbation and dry sex are discussed further in Chapter 6 of TEENS Sex AND CHOICES under "Risky Behavior."

27. How can I warn my child about sexual abusers?

Talking about sex can be difficult. Talking about sexual abuse is not any easier, but both are important. Whether your children are closer to three or 18, you need to remind both your sons and daughters that no one has the right to touch them except for the rare exception of a doctor during a physical exam.

At the conclusion of a parent seminar a mother shared with me about how her little 7-year-old daughter was sexually abused by an 8th grade neighbor boy. Unfortunately, not only does the little girl have painful memories of the abuse, she also contracted genital herpes. As you will learn in Chapter 8 of TEENS Sex AND CHOICES, herpes is an incurable STD. This little girl may have painful sores off and on for the rest of her life as a result of the sexual abuse.

Chapter 10 of TEENS Sex AND CHOICES describes sexual abuse, rape, and date rape for your children. They will also learn what to do if they find themselves in any of these situations.

28. When should guidelines for dating be established?

When guidelines for dating are established early, they help eliminate future problems. A mother shared with me that when her daughter was about six-years-old she brought up the subject of dating. She asked her little girl, "Do you know what your Daddy and I are going to let you do when you are about sixteen?"

With great excitement and curiosity and little girl replied, "No, Mommy! What?"

"Well," her mother responded, "When you are about sixteen, and *if* you prove to us you can make very wise choices, your father and I are going to let you start dating." The little girl's eyes glistened with excitement as she thought of her Prince Charming coming to take her on this wonderful date.

Throughout the next few years, the mother and daughter talked about what a fun date might be. When they saw teenagers together, they would discuss which couples looked like they were having fun and in a healthy relationship and which ones didn't look so healthy.

When the daughter was in the 8th grade, she came bouncing down the stairs all excited and announced that a young man had just invited her to go to a movie. The mother lovingly turned to her daughter and said, "You know, dear, I've been telling you for a long time that you would be able to date someday, but not before you were sixteen."

She said her daughter was disappointed over her response. She was even a little mad, but she was not surprised. Perhaps the path this wise mother began to pave when her daughter was six alleviated some of the frustration and pain for both mother and daughter.

You might try what a clever father told me he did with his grade-school-aged daughter. He explained that he frequently dates his daughter. That's right, he actually calls her on the telephone and invites her out. They set the time, place and activity together. The evening of the date he goes to his own house and rings his doorbell. His daughter greets him at the door dressed in the appropriate attire for the date. He then escorts her to the car and graciously opens her door.

"I treat my daughter like a princess on our dates," the father explained. "Just the way I expect other young men to do in years to come. I'm trying to set an example for my daughter. Future suitors will have to be extremely creative on dates to hold my daughter's attention. After all, she's used to being treated like royalty on her dates!"

A mother shared that she and her son also go on dates together. This all started when he was about 10. Since he didn't have enough money in his allowance, his mother would give him the money for the meal before they left the house. Once they arrived at the restaurant, they would look over the menu and the mother would tell her son what she would like. He then placed the order for both of them, paid the bill, left the tip, and escorted his mother back to the car.

The mother went on to tell me that her son is now 17 and they still go on dates. The only difference is that now they take *his car*. And recently when they were about to leave the house, he handed his mother a long stemmed rose.

These are examples of parents who are taking the time to teach their children what healthy dating is all about, long before dating begins. If you are not teaching them, where will they ever learn the etiquette of dating?

As you set guidelines for dating, keep in mind that it is easier to loosen the rules as you go along than tighten the reins once a young person starts dating. But don't get too rigid with your rules; this could lead to rebellion.

29. Do kids really date today?

No, not the way we used to. Perhaps your dating experiences were like mine. Before we were married, Chuck would pick me up each Friday and Saturday night and take me to a movie or dinner and then a movie. We would either double date or go out by ourselves. And of course Chuck always paid for all the dates.

But today things have changed. Kids seem to just hang out together in groups. That actually sounds good because what could go wrong in a crowd? Plenty, I assure you. Teenagers seem to always know whose parents are out of town or whose parents are "cool" and don't care what they do. After all, with 2,739 pregnancies and 8,219 STDs occurring among teenagers every day in America something is going on somewhere![7,8]

Before you rush to lock your children in a closet and throw away the key, let me make a very important point . . . *Not all teenagers are having sex!* In fact, the Centers for Disease Control recently announced that most teens across America are choosing abstinence. This is a reverse of a 40-year trend of rising sexual activity among U.S. high school students.[9]

Young people who grow up in a home feeling loved and appreciated and who have guidelines for dating are far less likely to become sexually active. The last two chapters of TEENS Sex AND CHOICES helps teens think about how to have fun dates without becoming physically involved.

30. When should young people start dating?

Statistics indicate the earlier young people begin to date the greater the chance they will become sexually active. In his book, *How to Help Your Child Say 'No' to Sexual Pressure,* Josh McDowell states,

> 91% of all girls who start dating at 12 have sex before graduation.
> 56% of all girls who start dating at 13 have sex before graduation.
> 53% of all girls who start dating at 14 have sex before graduation.
> 40% of all girls who start dating at 15 have sex before graduation.
> 20% of all girls who start dating at 16 have sex before graduation.

In other words, the longer you can postpone dating, the better off your child will be.

It's difficult to convince children that waiting another year or two is best. After all, a year is forever to a young person. But if you help them understand that they have a long life in front of them and help them establish additional goals other than finding a girlfriend or boyfriend, they may be more receptive.

Diligently work to make your home a fun and enjoyable place for your child. During the time before and even after he or she is allowed to date, you should provide alternatives to dating. Work on establishing a hobby together. Try taking a class together on karate, scuba diving, photography, or tennis. Have fun playing games together, going on picnics, going to the zoo, fishing, hunting, shopping, going to the show, ball games, and out to eat. Be creative and find activities your child enjoys. A young person sitting at home alone and bored on Friday and Saturday nights will not be a happy camper for long and may quickly turn into a rebellious teenager.

31. What about 12- to 14-year-olds going to the show together?

If a boy and girl go to the show together on a Saturday afternoon, this is considered by most people to be a date. Do you really want your 12, 13, or 14 year-old dating? Let me share a few true stories on this subject.

At the conclusion of a parent seminar, a mother told me a 7th grade boy asked her 7th grade daughter to the show. The mother was caught off guard and wasn't quite sure how to respond. (She obviously had not thought through guidelines for dating.) She knew the boy's mother and knew he came from a good family. After contemplating the situation for a moment, she determined it would be okay since this was just two kids going to an afternoon movie. What could it hurt?

The boy's mother came to pick her daughter up. When the daughter got home she was all excited and announced that during the movie the boy kissed her. The mother was surprised. She hadn't thought about that happening. But that first kiss was going to happen at some point, so she determined there was nothing to be concerned about.

A few weeks later the boy asked her daughter to go to the show again. Once again, the mother was caught off guard. (She still hadn't set any guidelines.) Should she allow this to keep going? She had said yes once before and she couldn't really come up with a good reason to say no now. This time her daughter came home even more excited than the first outing. "Mommy! You won't believe it. He kissed me over and over throughout the entire movie!"

The mother looked at me after sharing the story and asked, "Do you think we have started something a little too early?" Yes! I believe this is way too early. Think about it. This young 7th grade girl is now very excited and comfortable with kissing passionately. What's next? Is she going to be content stopping at passionate kissing for the next five years or will she be ready to touch under clothes and remove clothes in the near future? My guess is kissing will be boring real soon! Would you want your son going out with her?

Suggestion: If your child wants to go to the show with the opposite sex, go with them. Sit with them or near them. But don't drop them off at a dark theater all alone.

WARNING: A policeman in the Highland Park area of Dallas (upper class America) told me he was amazed how many parents drop their children, 12 to 15 years-old, off at the movie. As soon as the parents drive away, he said the kids walk out of the movie and go to nearby apartments. He didn't know what the kids were doing at the apartments but he was sure their parents would not approve.

Another mother told me the following story about her son. She said he had his first girlfriend in the 6th grade. The mom thought the little girl was cute and was pleased that her son had taken a liking to such a sweet little girl. One Saturday they invited the little girl to go to the zoo. The three of them had a great time looking at the animals and having a picnic. A few days later the mother was cleaning her son's bedroom and found a note from the little girl. Like any normal mother of a 6th grader, she sat down and read the note. It started out as a simple thank you for the fun trip to the zoo. Then the little girl concluded by saying, "but the most fun of all was sitting in the back seat of the car on the way home and playing with your penis."

The mother was horrified. She did not have a clue what was going on in the back seat on the way home. My question is this: Why was she promoting dating at such a young age in the first place? Why not ask one of the boys from school instead? I assure you the hormones will cause the attraction to the opposite sex to occur soon enough. Parents don't need to be encouraging dating at such a young age. It will happen soon enough all by itself.

Suggestion: If your child is not old enough to date and wants to ask a friend of the opposite sex to go somewhere, consider the "odd man rule." Let your child know that until he or she is old enough to date, there must be an odd number involved in the outing when the opposite sex is involved – like 1 boy and 2 girls or 3 boys and 2 girls. This will *help* eliminate pairing off. Then make sure you are able to keep an eye on them.

One last story along these lines: A principal of a Dallas elementary school recently told me she retrieved a note a 6th grade girl had written a 6th grade boy. Now keep in mind both of these were among the school's top students from good homes. The note simply said, "I really like you, and I want to do it with you. Don't worry if you don't have a condom, I have Saran Wrap."

Even the best of kids need supervision!

32. What about school dances for younger students?

I'm going to step on some toes here (no pun intended), but I think you should think twice about having school dances for younger students. Schools are working hard to prevent teenage pregnancies and sexual activity and yet they are encouraging 12-and 13-year-olds to get comfortable holding someone of the opposite sex as they sway to music. What's wrong with this picture?

Dances at an early age put a strain on young people. Although schools usually stress that the students do not have to have a date to attend the dance, many students do not heed that message. The stress over worrying about if someone will ask me to go, will someone ask me to dance once I'm there, or what if everyone laughs at the way I dance is really tough for these young people. It's hard enough for high school students to deal with such pressures, so why are we subjecting vulnerable 12- and 13-year-olds to this?

Another problem resulting from dances for younger students goes back to establishing rules for dating. The first guideline many parents establish is – no dating until you are 16. Should these parents make an exception for school dances? No doubt the child is going to say, "But everyone is going to the dance." After all, it is a school function. Either these parents are going to have to stick to their rules and take grief from their child or break their rules they've worked so hard to establish.

Suggestion – If you are going to hold a school party for younger students, get creative and come up with activities that don't require boys and girls pairing off and putting bodies together. Children are growing up fast enough and school dances only accelerate this process.

33. My child is interested in someone older. Is that a problem?

Yes, it definitely could be. It would be wise to let your child grow up knowing they will only be able to date people close to their own age. I would recommend teenagers date people within one year of their own age. Let's face it, the maturity and mindset of a 14-year-old-girl is very different from an 18-year-old boy.

Studies are indicating that the majority of teenage pregnancies are resulting from relationships with men 20 years of age or older. Many states are now enforcing laws that prohibit sex between adults and minors. Although these acts may be voluntary, they are often the result of manipulation by the older individual. State laws regarding this criminal offense vary from state to state.[10]

Although sexual activity and pregnancies can occur among young people of the same age, the odds go up drastically as the age gap increases. According to a report published by the California Department of Health Services:

- Men 20 years old and older father five times more births among junior high school aged girls than do junior high school aged boys.

- On average, when a 12-year-old or younger girl becomes pregnant, the father of the baby averages 22 years of age. When junior high aged girls become pregnant, the fathers of the babies are usually five years older than the mothers. When high school aged girls become pregnant, the fathers average nearly four years older.[11]

The age gap is not always between older men and younger girls. A principal of a rural junior high and high school told me they had a real problem with the high school girls seducing the junior high aged boys. This was a game the girls were playing and it was taking place inside and outside the school. It had become such a problem that the faculty had to monitor the halls during classes and lunch. Needless to say, the boys loved the attention from the older girls, but this was not a healthy situation for anyone concerned.

It will be extremely difficult or perhaps impossible to convince your 13-year-old daughter that this 20-year-old man is not good for her or that the relationship between your 14-year-old son and his 17-year-old girlfriend is not healthy. This is just one more reason why you need to establish guidelines *before these situations arise.* Not that having guidelines will automatically eliminate such problems, but it may help your child think through the situation before proceeding and it will prevent you from being caught off guard.

This is also one more reason why your home needs to be fun. A child who is secure at home, who has a close relationship with his or her parents and who greatly respects Mom and Dad will be less likely to be attracted to someone much older.

34. Is there a connection between alcohol and teen sexual activity?

Yes. According to a study published in the *Journal of Marriage and the Family,* the top risk factor for teens having sex is alcohol followed by a steady boyfriend or girlfriend, no parental monitoring, and having parents who think that adolescent sex is acceptable.[12]

A study by the Center of Addiction and Substance Abuse at New York's Columbia University found that:

- Sixty percent of college women who acquire STDs, including herpes and AIDS, were drunk at the time of infection.
- Ninety percent of rapes that occur on campus happen when alcohol is used by the perpetrator, the victim, or both.[13]

You will need to decide how you will deal with alcohol in your own home for you and your children. For example, some parents who have a glass of wine with dinner will occasionally allow their children to also have a glass of wine. That is a decision each family will need to make. However, I do not believe any parent has the right to make that decision for other parents. Let's face it, it is against the law for teenagers to drink. Therefore, it is wrong for parents to allow a party in their home where beer or other alcoholic beverages are served to minors.

Many parents justify their actions by taking the attitude that it is better for teens to drink in the safety of a home than out away from adult supervision. I question how much adult supervision is actually taking place and how many of the teens have their parents' permission to be drinking – probably not many, if any.

The point is abstinence and alcohol do not mix. One requires self-control while the other destroys it. It is important you let your child know exactly where you stand on the subject of drinking and drugs. The last chapter of TEENS Sex AND CHOICES addresses the subject of drugs and alcohol.

35. What about dating someone of a different race, religion, or economic background?

As written in the Constitution, all men are created equal. One of the great things about so many American children today is their blindness to racism. While you want to be careful not to cause your child to become racist, you do need to carefully consider your personal feelings about your child marrying someone of a different race, religion, or economic background. Some couples have gone into marriage with these differences and faced few problems. Others, however, never successfully overcome their differences.

If you have concerns about these issues, you would be wise to carefully explain to your child that marriage, even in the best of situations, requires hard work. When two people come from different backgrounds, this can result in added problems to the marriage and for their children. Using an illustration of a family member or friend who has experienced these problems might help.

For example, a lady shared with me that she grew up Baptist and she married a Catholic. While they were dating, religion was far from their thoughts. After the wedding and a few children, religion became a major issue. Determining which church to raise their children in became a source of on going frustration in their marriage.

Keep in mind that it will be almost impossible for a young person to see your point of view if he or she is already in the serious relationship. That is why these guidelines should be established long before your child becomes emotionally involved with another person. Adding new rules in the midst of a dating relationship will nearly always result in rebellion. On the other hand, a child who is raised from a young age with the concept of dating and marrying someone of similar background will be more likely to embrace this concept as a family value, not as one more rigid rule from Mom and Dad.

36. What about curfews?

Set a *reasonable* time for both your sons and daughters to come home on weekends and school nights. Personally, I would think long and hard about letting a high school student stay out after midnight. What possible good can come from teenagers being out that late?

A 14-year-old girl who had been in all kinds of trouble with the police told me her mother had recently set a nightly curfew. When I asked how she felt about these new rules, she smiled and said, "In a strange way, it feels good. For the first time I think maybe my mother cares about me."

It would also be wise to require your children to keep you posted on what they are doing and where they are going. Make sure they agree to call if they see they are going to be late or their plans change.

Suggestion: *You* need to set the example for your children. Always let your family know where you can be reached and what time you plan to be home. Call if you are running late and let them know what time they can expect you. If you always do this for them, they will not feel offended if you require the same of them. This will just become a simple courtesy your family always provides for each other.

37. Does anyone set limits on the telephone anymore? What about girls calling boys?

Somewhere in parenting we have lost the knack of passing on telephone etiquette. One of the most frustrating issues I hear parents discussing today is what to do about the telephone. Whether it's a 12-year-old girl calling boys after school or a 17-year-old boy calling girls after midnight, the telephone is a major problem!

Many parents have resolved the problem by installing a private line for their children. While that may take care of the problems in their home, it doesn't resolve the problems their child causes for the families he or she is calling. Let's face it, there is nothing worse than waking up at 2:00 a.m. to a ringing phone. Your heart pounds as you are trying to prepare yourself for who might have just died. Then when you recognize the voice on the other end as a teenage boy asking to speak to your daughter, you don't know whether to be relieved or angry.

Whether you have a son or daughter, you need to teach your children telephone etiquette. These rules should be established as soon as your child starts using the phone and be regularly adjusted to fit the child's age. Rules should include time limits and time frames. Keep in mind that it is always easier to loosen rules than to tighten them later.

The telephone, like television, has become another form of keeping children out of their parents' way. Parents feel that as long as their child is talking on the phone nothing can go wrong. With Call Waiting, many parents have done away with time limits. Parents need to ask themselves if this is wise use of their child's time. Is the conversation healthy and productive? Would reading a book, playing outside, establishing a hobby, or helping with dinner be more productive?

Establishing telephone rules will not only help your child show respect to your family, it will also ensure that your child is respecting the family members in the homes he or she is calling. Consider the following for a child in first through fourth grade:

1. No phone conversations until all homework is completed.
2. No more than 15 minutes on the phone a day.
3. No calls are to made or received after 7 p.m.

These rules provide limited phone privileges for young children. By allowing only 15 minutes each day, your child will begin to develop a decision making process. As soon as your child picks up the phone, the clock is ticking and a decision has to be made, "Is this how I want to spend a portion of my 15 minutes?" What a great way to help your child begin developing self-discipline!

Although the rules can be expanded as your child gets older, make sure you always have a time limit for when calls can be made and received in your home. Most adults would never consider calling a friend or business associate after 10:00 or 10:30 p.m. except for an emergency. Shouldn't we teach our children to observe the same guidelines? This is merely a matter of respect; respect for all family members on both ends of the line.

Girls calling boys - The number one complaint I hear from parents of boys is that girls are calling their sons at all hours of the day and night. By the time your child starts school, you need to decide where you stand when it comes to girls calling boys and how you will deal with this issue. As early as first and second grade girls are calling boys, and it only gets worse through the grade school and junior high ages. Whether your child is the one doing the calling or receiving the calls, you have the right to set rules and expect them to be observed. Let's look at both sides and then you can decide how you will deal with this dilemma.

If you are opposed to your daughter calling boys, there's nothing wrong with keeping the same rule most of us were raised with long, long ago: Girls do not call boys except for rare exceptions or emergencies. Many parents are sticking with this rule and successfully passing it on to their daughters. If you go this route, just make sure you provide a logical explanation for your stand.

However, if you allow your daughter to call boys, please inform her that most parents do not appreciate girls who do all the calling. If the boy never calls her, that probably means she is far more interested in him than he is in her. You might want to tell her that she is not to call a boy unless he is also calling her. This will help prevent your daughter from chasing after boys and becoming a nuisance to both the boy and his family. Make sure you establish and enforce time limits and time frames when your daughter can use the phone.

If you are one of those frustrated parents who's life has been turned upside down because girls are calling your son at all hours of the day and night, stop the madness by establishing some rules. After all, boys also need time limits and time frames. As you set these rules you can decide how you will deal with on going calls from girls.

The following are a couple of ideas parents have told me they have successfully tried. Several parents have said they just make a point of answering the phone each time it rings. When a girl asks for their son, they simply tell her that it is their family policy that girls are not to call boys. They ask for her name and number and inform her that their son will return her call if he wishes to talk to her. It is then up to their son whether he wants to return her call or not. It doesn't take long before she catches on and stops the annoying phone calls.

Other parents have said they have told their son that when a girl calls, he may talk to her for 5 minutes. If he wants to continue to talk to her, he must hang up and call her back. This helps the girl respect his family values. If he doesn't want to talk to her, he can just tell her he can't talk right now.

Remember, this is your phone. You pay the bills. You have a right to expect your children and their friends to respect your rules.

38. Is it important to always know who your child is dating?

What would you do if a teenage boy, who was a total stranger, rang your doorbell and asked to borrow your brand new car for the evening? Even if he promised to return it by midnight, would you hand him the keys? I doubt it. Yet isn't it interesting that we will let total strangers come to the door and take our children out without any idea who they are.

Suggestion: Find creative ways of meeting the person your child is dating. Have them over for dinner, play cards, go out for pizza . . . whatever. Surely, your child is more important to you than a car.

In our home, my husband always had a rule that every young man who took our daughters out had to come to the house and meet him. As each new suitor came to the door, Chuck simply let him know that his daughters were very precious to him and he expected him to bring his daughter home in better condition than she left. I'm not sure if it was my husband's 6'4" 250 pound stature or the way he spoke to the young men, but they definitely seemed to get the message.

39. Do I need to wait up for my children? They're good kids!

If you ever hear me speak at a parent seminar, I can almost guarantee you will hear me stress this point. I believe every child across America needs a mom and/or dad waiting up when they come home at night. Whether it is your 6-year-old coming home from a birthday party or your 18-year-old coming in from a date or a night out with some buddies, I challenge you to wait up. Get into a habit of greeting your child at the door with a smile on your face and enthusiastically saying, "What did you do tonight? Who'd you see?" Let your children grow up knowing you will always be waiting up for them.

Parents have asked, "But if I wait up, doesn't that make my child think I don't trust him?" Probably so – if you greet your child with a stern face and say something like, "What did you do wrong tonight?" But if you are smiling and act enthusiastic to hear all the details of the evening there should be no feelings of distrust.

There are several reasons why waiting up is so important. First, you will never get more information about the evening's events than when your child first walks in the door. If the evening was exciting, how great that Mom and/or Dad is there to hear the great news. If the evening was a disaster, how great that Mom and/or Dad is there to listen and provide solace.

A 20-year-old told me her father always waited up for her when she was a teenager. Now that she is in college, her father doesn't make curfews an issue anymore. He considers her an adult and trusts her. He does, however, continue to wait up for her. She has told him on numerous occasions that it isn't necessary to wait up for her any longer. He just smiles and says he just sleeps better knowing she's home safely. As a result, she works hard to always be home at a reasonable time out of respect for her father.

A mother told me she left one of my parent seminars determined to start waiting up for her 16-year-old daughter. She said she was amazed what that did for their relationship. Although the waiting up part was hard, she said just being there for her daughter has completely changed their relationship!

Here's another reason to wait up for your child: if a teenager knows Mom or Dad will be waiting up when they walk in the door, he will think long and hard about getting involved in drugs and alcohol. Even if he does get involved, you will be in a much better position to catch the early signs if you have a conversation with him when he walks in the door.

Now let me share my own personal reason for encouraging you to wait up for your children. My husband and I are convinced if our parents had waited up for us when we were dating, it would have made all the difference in the outcome of our lives. (I share my own story in chapter 4 of TEENS Sex AND CHOICES.) I only had one rule when I was dating: I had to be home at 11 o'clock on Friday and Saturday night. And every Friday and Saturday I walked in the door at 11 o'clock. But I also knew all I had to do was walk in and lock the door, turn off the light, and walk down a dark hallway. You see at my house at 11 o'clock my parents were always in bed asleep – and I knew it.

But what a difference if Mom or Dad had been in the den watching television or reading a book. I can just imagine walking in the door and shouting out, "I'm home. See you in the morning." And then hearing one of my parents say, "Wait a minute, Marilyn. Come talk to me for a minute." Then I walk in the den, look at my mother or father's smiling face and hear them say, "What did you and Chuck do tonight?" THINK ABOUT IT!

There is no way I could have looked my parents square in the eye after having sex 20 minutes before. It just couldn't have happened! Here's another thought. If my parents had waited up for me, I think they would have caught on early in the relationship that something was happening. You see I didn't look as nice in the evening when I came home as I did when I left. My face was flushed, my hair was messed up, not to mention my clothes being a wrinkled mess. These signs would have been easily noticed had someone been waiting up for me.

40. How can I encourage my children to wait until marriage?

When conducting a parent seminar, I give parents three key sentences to say to their children. I believe when a child grows up hearing these three sentences over and over it makes a huge impact on the outcome of their life. The three sentences are:

1. I love you!
2. I'm proud of you!
3. I don't want you to have sex until you get married!

Chuck and I believe that if our parents had waited up for us and said over and over, "I love you. I'm proud of you. And I don't want you to have sex until you get married" that we would not have had sex before we were married. You see we were two really good kids who came from really good homes. But the best of kids from the best of homes need guidance, direction, and protection.

Once your child is in a relationship, I recommend you talk to both of them. Chuck and I think our parents would have been wise to have talked to both of us once they realized we were getting serious. The talk could have gone something like this: "Chuck – Marilyn, we're glad you're having fun going out together, but we want you to know that we do not want there to be any physical activity going on between the two of you. Chuck, we expect you to treat our daughter with respect. Marilyn, we do not want you coming on to Chuck."

I'm sure Chuck and I would have been embarrassed by such a talk, but we are also convinced we would have listened if someone had made the effort to talk to us.

By the way, who's talking to your children?

41. My child doesn't like my hugs anymore. Should I stop?

Studies have proven babies who are not held at birth often become sick, weak, and even die. Babies obviously need physical love. But when does this craving cease? At what age does a person stop needing this display of affection? Personally, I don't think it ever ends.

My husband has learned after thirty years of marriage there are times I need a hug. He might be in his chair watching television or on the couch reading a book and suddenly I crawl in his lap and snuggle in his arms. It took many years for him to learn that this is not necessarily a sexual come-on. Sometimes it simply means, "Marilyn needs a hug." He places his arms around me, holds me for a few minutes, and within moments I walk away with an overwhelming sense of contentment. Now if a woman in her forties needs to be held from time to time, how much more do our sons and daughters need to be held?

Many children love to be hugged throughout their lives. Others seem to reject it after a while. Our daughters were perfect examples of both cases. Shannan, our older daughter, has let us hug her all her life. Windi, on the other hand, started out as our more affectionate child and then went through a stage around the sixth or seventh grade where it wasn't cool for Mom and Dad to hug her. Perhaps you have experienced this with your children. We would go to hug her and she would go limp, like a wet wash rag. Perhaps it was the stubbornness in me, but I determined to keep hugging my daughter despite her rejection. I even told her once, "Maybe you don't need my hugs anymore, but I still need to hold you." I was careful not to hug her in public, but at home the hugs continued.

Within time Windi changed her attitude as she began to hug us back. (It feels so good!) And now even though she is a wife and mother, we do lots of hugging when we are together. I love the warmth of my daughter's arms around me. I only hope it gives her half the satisfaction it brings to me. I shudder to think how close we came to ending this intimate part of our relationship.

42. Should a father hug his teenage children?

No matter how successful we might become in life, we all want acceptance from our parents. Hugs shout acceptance! Teens struggle enough with their self-image, self-confidence, and inadequacies without thinking their own parents don't accept them.

When it comes to hugs, there is just something natural about a mother hugging her children. It seems to be second nature. But unfortunately, in a day where sexual abuse is sweeping our society, many fathers are apprehensive to show affection to their children. The truth of the matter is, Fathers, your children need your hugs! Your sons and your daughters need your affection.

I encourage you to find special times to pat your son on the back. At other times let go and give him a big, old, loving bear hug. Let him know you love him both by your words and actions.

Now, about your daughters; Dads, I challenge you to tenderly hug and hold your little girls. Let them know you are there to love and protect them. Your gentle embrace should serve as a constant reminder that you will always be there for her. Remember, if you are not the one holding your little girl, she might try to find someone else to fill that need. So as her father, lovingly hug her. And please do not stop the hugs until you take her hand and walk her down the aisle and entrust her to that young man on her wedding day. (But even then, don't stop hugging her. After all even married women like to feel their father's hugs!)

At the conclusion of an adult seminar, a lady shared with me that her father suddenly stopped hugging her when she was about twelve years old. For years she kept asking herself what she did that was so bad that her dad would suddenly stop hugging her. Perhaps this father felt that since his little girl was turning into a young lady it was no longer appropriate for him to hug her. If only this father could have determined in his mind that these gestures were non-sexual and really necessary for his daughter's well being. If he were unable to bring his thoughts under control, no doubt it would be better to stop the physical contact than to allow these emotions to get out of hand. His gentle smile and a soft pat on the shoulder could still have proven to be encouraging to his daughter.

In his book, *Raising Positive Kids in a Negative World,* Zig Ziglar refers to Dr. Ross Campbell, a psychiatrist who specializes in working with children. Dr. Campbell states that in all his reading and experience, he has never known of one sexually disoriented person who had a warm, loving, and affectionate father.

As a word of caution, if you have not been hugging your children on a regular basis, don't suddenly smother them with hugs and kisses. This sudden change in behavior could cause great alarm for all those concerned! Instead, you might begin with a casual pat on the back and gradually build up to a genuine hug. If your child seems to resist, don't give up. Take it slow and give him or her time to get used to it.

43. My child's father is not on the scene. What should I do?

A single mom needs to be sure her children interact with men of strong character. I am amazed how many 13- and 14-year-old girls have told me they never intend to marry. When I ask them to tell me about their father, they usually say they haven't seen their dad for months or years. A loving grandfather, uncle or friend whom you trust and who holds your same values may not be able to replace Dad, but he is definitely better than no male role model or male affirmation.

You might also find other positive male role models in scout troops, church youth groups, team sports and other youth organizations.

44. With all the sex and violence on TV, what guidelines should be set?

How much time do you spend each week with your child – talking, playing games, cooking, working together on a project or hobby? How does that amount of time compare to the time your child spends watching TV? Unfortunately, television often starts off as a convenient baby sitter when children are young, then it gradually replaces Mom and Dad during the teenage years.

According to a report from Nielson Media Research, children from 2 to 11 watch 23 hours of television per week. By the time the average child leaves elementary school, he or she has witnessed 8,000 murders and 100,000 other acts of violence on the television screen. By the time the average child graduates from high school, he has spent approximately 12,000 hours in the classroom and more than 18,000 hours in front of the television set.[14]

I encourage you to set a limit on how much time the TV set can be viewed each day. I would also set guidelines as to what type of shows you and your children watch. Think about this: Would you let some total strangers come into your house to have hot passionate sex in your living room while your children watched? I'm sure your answer is NO! So why do most parents let Hollywood bring gorgeous actors into their home every day on TV to do the same thing and not think anything about it? Sure TV is not real life, but do children understand that?

If you have small children, I recommend you be very careful about the shows you watch when they are awake. An 18-year-old boy recently told me he learned all about sex in his living room when he was five-years-old. He said he would play with his toys in the middle of the room while his parents watched soap operas. His parents didn't realize he was capable of playing with his toys while paying close attention to what was happening on TV. If a child can learn that much from soap operas, think what R-rated videos do.

45. What are some recommended guidelines for movies?

It is important to set some standards about what types of movies your child can and cannot see. Unfortunately, you can't always go by the rating of the movie. This past weekend my husband and I went to a comedy that was rated PG-13. The theater was filled with kids of all ages. Thirty minutes into the movie we got up and walked out. Sex was the primary subject matter and the women were scantily clothed (close to being nude.) As we left the theater, I wondered how many parents thought they were sending their children to a family type movie simply because it was rated PG-13.

Suggestion: Don't trust ratings. Talk to others who have seen the movie or go see it yourself. Set standards for your children and challenge them to walk out of movies that don't meet your family's standards. (That isn't easy for most teens.)

Don't hand money over week after week for your child's entertainment. Make them pay for their own entertainment either from their job or allowance. When our girls were teenagers, Chuck and I felt we were being bled to death each weekend as we handed five and ten dollar bills over for their entertainment. Today you're probably handing over twenty-dollar bills. If you have two or three children, that can add up to some serious money! Chuck and I finally put a stop to this by giving our girls a set amount of money each month. If they ran out of money by the end of the month, playtime was over. This really caused them to think carefully about where they went and how they were spending their money.

Use this opportunity to help your children become movie critics. Require they share at least three good things about the movie as well as three bad things. This can make for great dinner time discussions. Ask your children to discuss the values the movie was promoting. Were the actors drinking, doing drugs, and smoking in the movie? Were there any negative consequences to these actions? (Probably not.) Was there sexual content to the movie? (Probably so.) Was it within marriage or outside marriage? What was the underlying message of this movie?

Have fun with these discussions and don't let them turn into heated arguments. You simply want to train your children to think during a movie as opposed to mindlessly soaking in whatever Hollywood is trying to promote.

46. What about kids taking the opposite sex into their bedrooms?

A mother recently told me her 16-year-old daughter had a 17-year-old boyfriend. Being impressed with both the young man and his family, the mother had no problem when her daughter began spending more and more time at his house. After all, they were just playing computer games and watching TV. Initially, this sounded healthy and safe until the mother found out the computer and VCR were in the boy's bedroom.

Taking into consideration these were two good kids did this mother really have anything to be concerned about? Of course she did, because good has nothing to do with it. Good kids from good homes still have raging hormones. Watching a movie while sitting or lying on a bed, leaning up against a bed or merely looking at the bed from across the room can be very suggestive. Parents who allow this are really encouraging their children to get comfortable with yet one more step toward intimacy.

Parents need to provide a place for their children to entertain their friends of the opposite sex that is not a bedroom and is not secluded from the rest of the family.

47. How have we gotten where we are today?

America is becoming desensitized. If you watch sex on TV and in movies long enough you accept it as normal. If you let your teenage son take his date into his bedroom long enough, you'll eventually get comfortable with the idea. When he begins to shut the door behind them, it may bother you at first, but give it a little more time. You'll get comfortable with that as well.

A 17-year-old girl told me she was in the school play. Being the leading lady, she had to make a number of quick costume changes. She said it was not unusual to run behind the stage and grab the first available person to unzip her dress. If that person happened to be a stagehand or the leading man, it didn't matter. All that mattered was that the dress came off quickly and the next one went on. In other words, forget modesty – the show must go on! She said the first time one of the guys helped her get out of her dress she felt a little uncomfortable, but after a while it became no big deal.

The internet is another way Americans are becoming desensitized. How easy it is for your child to look through pornographic material free of charge or go into a chat room and start talking to a total stranger. If the conversation in the chat room becomes sexual, it doesn't matter because the person your child is talking to can't tell how uncomfortable or embarrassed your child is. Besides, give it a few more tries and your child will get good at this. Of course, once your child becomes comfortable talking in a chat room it will be far easier to have such discussions face to face.

Suggestion: Keep TVs, VCRs and computers in a room where you can monitor what is going on.

Teach your children, *starting at a young age*, right from wrong! Don't just cop out and say it's wrong "because I said so." Explain why it is wrong and expect your child to do what is right. Let's face it, you will probably not be around the first time your child is offered drugs, asked to have sex, or watch a pornographic movie. How will your child know if these are wrong unless you have taken the time to teach him right from wrong? He must buy into the concept and understand the risks to his dreams and goals.

TEENS Sex AND CHOICES will provide you numerous opportunities to share your values on such issues as drugs, alcohol, sex, and pornography without embarrassment.

48. What about girl-boy slumber parties?

Girl-boy slumber parties are becoming quite popular today. If this is a party where activities are going on all night and is well chaperoned from beginning to end, then I think an occasional girl-boy all night party is okay. If, however, the object is to have fun until one or two o'clock in the morning and then everyone is going to find a couch, a chair or location on the floor to curl up and go to sleep – I don't think it is smart. What possible good can come from such events?

How can parents say they are concerned about reducing teen pregnancies and sexual activity while they are helping teenagers get comfortable sleeping next to each other? Even if the boys go in one room and the girls go in another room to sleep, it's pretty exciting to think your boyfriend or girlfriend is sleeping in the next room. Teenagers have raging hormones and they don't need lots of help to get their imaginations running wild.

Suggestion: These parties are so popular today that I can almost guarantee you will be facing this issue. You would be wise to share with your children how you plan to deal with this before it ever comes up.

Anytime your children ask if they can go to a slumber party, ask if there will be boys and girls attending. No matter how they answer, you would be smart to find out all the circumstances surrounding the party including adult supervision and whether or not those adults share your values. If it is a girl-boy all night party, find out what sleeping arrangements have been made and whether alcohol will be served.

49. Don't I run the risk of my children lying to me if I don't let them do what everyone else is doing?

Any parent who establishes rules for their children runs the risk of rebellion. If you tell your 4-year-old that she can't have a piece of candy before dinner, she may sneak behind your back and take a piece anyway. Does that mean you shouldn't have made the rule? No. It simply means you need to clearly explain why she can't have the candy and then be prepared with a punishment if she disobeys. If the punishment is appropriately administered, she will learn a valuable lesson. If the punishment wasn't severe enough, she will find more clever ways of taking the candy so you won't catch her next time.

It is the same with your teenager. If you tell your daughter she cannot go to a boy-girl slumber party because it goes against your family values, you run the risk that next time she will just lie about the situation. If you catch her in a lie, you need to stay calm and don't yell. Yelling will do more harm than good. First let her know that even though you are deeply disappointed in her choices, that you still love her very much. Talk to her and make sure she understands why her actions were wrong. Then determine a suitable punishment. It needs to be severe enough that she will feel regret and remorse and never want to go through that punishment again.

Do you see why it is so important to teach young children values? If a boy learns it is wrong to lie to his parents when he is 5-years-old, he may be compelled to tell the truth the rest of his life. If, on the other hand, he gets away with lying at five, he may end up being a perpetual liar the rest of his life. The same is true with stealing, cheating, and being disrespectful of others.

50. What if my child asks, "So, Mom, Dad – Did you wait until you were married?"

The greatest fear most parents face in talking to their children about sex is the inevitable question, "So, Mom, Dad, did you have sex before you were married?" Dreading this question is no reason to avoid the subject. There are some rather easy solutions.

If you did wait, be prepared to share how you succeeded at this lifestyle. Talk about the boundaries you set as well as the frustrations and struggles you faced while waiting. Talk about the peer pressure you dealt with and the benefits you enjoy now because of your *CHOICES*.

If you did not wait, I encourage you to be honest with your children. But you don't need to tell them all the details. You can answer your child's question by simply saying, "You know, I made some mistakes along these lines when I was growing up. But back when I was growing up no one was talking about sex and the consequences weren't all that serious. Today, the consequences can be life threatening. And today, I'm talking to you. I believe you are capable of being more successful than I was."

By sharing this information you didn't tell your child what you did or did not do. The intimate details are not necessary and are really none of their business.

Some parents who did not wait until marriage feel hypocritical asking their children to postpone sex. But ask yourself the following questions: Did you ever play in the street as a small child? Did you ever steal some candy? Did you ever cheat on a test? Did you ever drive at excessive speeds? Did you ever drink while underage or experiment with drugs?

If you answer yes to one or more of these questions, are you a hypocrite if you don't give full approval for your child to play in the street, steal, cheat, speed, or become involved in drugs and alcohol? No, you aren't a hypocrite, you are a wise parent who wants the best for your child!

As you are about to learn, the circumstances of sexual activity are drastically different today than ten, twenty, or thirty years ago. Parents who encourage their children to postpone sex today are not hypocritical. They are loving, wise parents.

References

[1] Thomson and Colella, University of Wisconsin-Madison, 1992.

[2] Bumpass, L.L., et al., "The Role of Cohabitation in Declining Rates of Marriage," *Journal of Marriage and the Family.* November 1991; 53, 913-928.

[3] Cunningham and Antill, Macquarie University, 1994.

[4] Resnick, Michael, D., Ph.D., et al., "Protecting Adolescents from Harm: Findings from the National Longitudinal Study on Adolescent Health," *Journal of the American Medical Association,* September 10, 1997.

[5] Ibid.

[6] Centers for Disease Control and Prevention. "Youth Risk Behavior Surveillance – United States, 1995. *Morbidity and Mortality Weekly Report,* September 1998; 47 (SS-3).

[7] The Alan Guttmacher Institute, "Teen Sex and Pregnancy," *Facts in Brief,* July 1996.

[8] Kaiser Family Foundation and American Social Health Association, *STDs in America: How Many Cases and At What Cost?* Menlo Park, CA, 1998.

[9] Centers for Disease Control and Prevention, Atlanta, GA, July 12, 1999.

[10] Maynard, R.A. (ed.). *Kids Having Kids: A Robin Hood Foundation Special Report on the Costs of Adolescent Childbearing.* New York: Robin Hood Foundation, 1996.

[11] California Department of Health Services, "California Residents' Live Births, 1990 by Age of Mother, Age of Father, Race, Marital Status," *California Vital Statistics Section – 1992.* Sacramento, CA.

[12] Small, S.A. & Luster, T., "Adolescent Sexual Activity: An Ecological Risk Factor Approach." *Journal of Marriage and the Family,* February, 1994; 56, 181-192.

[13] Center of Addiction and Substance Abuse (CASA), *Rethinking Rites of Passage: Substance Abuse on America's Campuses; A Report of the Commission on Substance Abuse at Colleges and Universities.* New York: Columbia University, 1994.

[14] Huston, A.C., University of Nebraska Press, *Big World, Small Screen: The Role of Television in American Society,* Lincoln, NE, 1992.

Chapter 4

Dealing with Tough Issues

The following is a list of issues you will be dealing with (or you may already be dealing with) as your children go through the teenage years. When dealing with teenagers it is wise to use the Boy Scout motto: Be Prepared. A wise parent will carefully consider these situations and have a ready answer before they arise. If you are married, it is important that you and your spouse come to an agreement on how to deal with each of these issues. Children don't need the added frustration of Mom and Dad having divergent opinions.

As you go through the list, remember what has already been stated numerous times – it is easier to loosen rules than to tighten the reins! Also realize some of your answers will never change, regardless of your child's age, while others will vary greatly depending on age.

1. Do your children know what you believe about sex before marriage? If yes, how do they know? If no, when and how do you plan to talk about this?

2. Can your children talk to you about sex and other personal issues? If yes, list some discussions you and your child have shared together. If no, what do you plan to do to open the doors of communication?

3. What are your beliefs about drugs, alcohol, and smoking? Do your children know and understand where you stand on these issues?

ABCs of the Birds and Bees

4. Do you and your child share several activities and hobbies together? If yes, what are they? If no, what do you plan to do about it?

5. Does your child know you love him/her? If yes, how? If no, what can you do to change this?

6. Does your child have positive male and female role models in his/her life? If yes, who are they? If no, what can you do to change this?

7. What are you going to do if your teenager wants to take someone of the opposite sex into his/her bedroom?

8. What will you do if your child wants to go to a show, a party, or school dance with someone of the opposite sex before he/she is allowed to date? Will it matter if they say they are just friends?

9. At what age will your child be allowed to date?

10. Will you have restrictions regarding the age difference of the people your child dates, their race, or religion? If yes, what are the restrictions and reasons?

11. Does your child understand and agree with your dating restrictions?

12. What will the curfew be for dating?

13. Will there be exceptions to the curfew? If so, what are some examples?

14. How do you plan to get to know the people your child dates?

15. How do you plan to deal with boy/girl slumber parties?

16. How do you plan to deal with school dances before your child is allowed to date?

17. Do you believe telephone rules are necessary? If so, what should they be?

18. Do you have limits or rules for TV? If so, what are they?

19. Do you have limits and rules for the internet? If so, what are they?

20. Do you have limits and rules for movies? If so, what are they?

21. Have you talked with your child about sexual abuse in the past year?

BOOK TWO

TEENS
Sex AND
CHOICES

PARENT EDITION

BOOK TWO

SECTION ONE

WOW! I DIDN'T KNOW THAT!

> Success requires
> Knowledge and Understanding

Note to Parents

This first chapter is designed to be fun. You will begin by guessing each other's dreams and goals. This will allow you to see how well you and your children know each other.

After you finish discussing dreams and goals, your children are going to ask you a few simple questions about where and when you learned about sex. This will be a great place to interject some humor. Did you learn by kids whispering on the playground? Did you and a friend sneak a book out of the house? A few funny stories can help break the tension you and your children might be feeling.

Your children are also going to ask you if you feel weird talking about sex with them. If you do, admit it. Make a joke about the fact that you plan on getting a lot better by the time you are finished with the series. If you are honest now, it will help your children be honest and open with you as the chapters progress.

The simple questions your children will be asking you are not designed to lead to personal questions about your past. If, however, your children ask personal questions at anytime during this series, you can either give them the answers to their questions or tell them you will answer their questions a little later in the Family Discussion. This will allow you to get more comfortable talking to your children and determine how much information you want to give. Review question #50 in Chapter 3 of this book, "What if my child asks, 'So, Mom, Dad – Did you wait until you were married?'" Remember, there is no need to ever give your children explicit details about your past unless you choose to do so. You are in control of the discussion. It is up to you how much or how little you tell them.

The Workbook assignment concludes with a pretest. This will give your family a glimpse of what lies ahead. All family members should take the test. The answers are in the back of the book. **DO NOT explain the correct answers to your children**. It will be much better for them to learn the answers for themselves as they continue through the series.

A Tip from the Tool Box:

> If you do most of the talking during the Family Discussions, you will never know what your child is thinking.

Chapter 1

CHOICES

CHOICES. You make them every day. Some are small and insignificant. Others will have a profound impact on the rest of your life. The bottom line is this: the *CHOICES* you make today can lead to success or serious regrets. The secret is learning how to make *CHOICES* that lead to lifelong success

This book is like a toolbox that can help you learn how to make *CHOICES* which will guide you toward success. As you learn to skillfully use the enclosed tools, you will be able to apply them to all areas of your life.

A topic has been carefully selected for this series that will serve as training in making wise *CHOICES*. I guarantee this is a topic that will interest all readers. I can also guarantee you are going to be dealing with *CHOICES* about this issue for the rest of your life. The decisions you make in this area can result in lifelong success or a lifetime of regrets.

What is this topic that is guaranteed to interest all readers? What else? . . . Sex!

The Journey Begins

As you begin this book you are embarking on a journey, perhaps one of the most unusual excursions of your life. This book is going to help you find the secret to *SENSATIONAL SEX!* – Hold it! Wait just a minute! Before you get carried away, this does not mean you are ready for sex right now, but one day you will be. And as you begin this search for *SENSATIONAL SEX,* you will face many decisions.

In fact, the *CHOICES* you make about sex will be among the most important decisions you will ever make in your life. But it will be impossible to make wise *CHOICES* without accurate information. That is why one of the most important tools you will be using in this series is the tool of knowledge and understanding.

Tool #1

> *CHOICES that Lead to Lifelong Success*
> require
> Knowledge and Understanding

Probably the most startling fact of all is that your parents or some other adult probably handed this book to you and asked you to read it. Well, get over the shock, because it's true. They really do want to help you learn to make *CHOICES* that lead to lifelong success which includes finding the secret to *SENSATIONAL SEX!*

How to Use This Material

Each participating family member should **read the book** or **listen to the tapes**. (The information is the same for both.) At the end of each chapter students will be instructed to complete their **workbook** exercises followed by the **Family Discussion**. This discussion will become another valuable tool as you and your parents talk, laugh, and share together.

From your parents' standpoint, it probably seems like only yesterday when they were your age. They really do understand raging hormones, peer pressure, and the desire to love and be loved. You might be surprised at the words of wisdom they will have to offer on this subject. That brings us to the second important tool:

Tool #2

CHOICES that Lead to Lifelong Success
require
Learning from Those with Experience

This series is filled with incredible facts and information which will astonish young and old alike. However, great effort was taken to make sure there is no embarrassment. So, whether you are a young person or an adult, relax and have fun as you learn together. Remember:

A family that can talk together about sex
can talk about *anything!*

Let the Search Begin . . .

It is a fact that humans gain a natural appetite for sex during the teenage years. This is a normal part of growing up. Your parents, grandparents, and all the generations before you have gone through this same sexual awakening. There is a big difference, however, between today's attitude regarding sex and yesteryear's.

Before the 1960s most people saved sex for marriage. Once married, the husband and wife would usually remain faithfully committed to each other throughout life. The divorce rate was low. Pregnancies among single girls were rare. There were only two significant sexually transmitted diseases (STDs), syphilis and gonorrhea. After penicillin became widely available in the 1940s there was no fear of people dying from a sexually transmitted disease.

Then came the sexual revolution of the 1960s. It promoted sexual freedom for young and old alike. Today, men and women of all ages indulge in sexual relationships outside of marriage without being judged or condemned. While the thought of sexual freedom may have sounded like a great idea, there was a slight glitch which few considered. The sexual freedom of the '60s produced a national epidemic of teenage pregnancies and a long list of sexually transmitted diseases. Many of these diseases have no cure and several are deadly.

Obviously, as you search for the secret to *SENSATIONAL SEX* you will want to make *CHOICES* which will help you avoid sexually transmitted diseases and unwanted pregnancies. Let's face it. Painful, disgusting sores resulting from STDs are not going to win you a prize as the world's greatest lover. So how do you achieve *SENSATIONAL SEX* while avoiding STDs and teenage pregnancies? That is a question you will have to answer for yourself as you work through this series. There are, however, two popular views for you to consider.

Two Possible Solutions

One possible solution encourages the safer sex message. Advocates of safer sex promote the use of condoms. The **condom** is a thin latex rubber covering that fits over a man's penis during sexual intercourse. Advocates claim that if the condom is used consistently and correctly every time a person has sex, it will prevent the spread of STDs and reduce the chances of a pregnancy.

The other possible solution is sexual abstinence until marriage. Advocates of **abstinence** believe the only guaranteed way to prevent teenage pregnancies and STDs is for two mutually **monogamous** people to remain faithfully committed to each other for life. Simply stated, that means two people who save sex exclusively for marriage. (You can check the glossary in the back of the book anytime you find an unfamiliar word, such as monogamous.)

It is your job to choose which one of these views will lead you to the secret of *SENSATIONAL SEX*. Condom advocates believe it is unrealistic for people to wait until marriage. Abstinence advocates say it is unrealistic to believe condoms provide enough protection. Wow! I'd say you have some tough *CHOICES* ahead of you!

I will admit I have strong convictions about these two views, but I'm not going to tell you which one I believe is best until later in the book. At that time you will also learn why I have devoted my life to speaking with teenagers on this subject. Throughout this book I will present accurate information on both views so you can choose for yourself which one is best for you.

Remember, you are not going to make *CHOICES* that lead to lifelong success unless you have knowledge and understanding. Have fun as you and your family learn to talk together about this super sensational subject!

At this time complete **Workbook Chapter 1** beginning on the following page.

Thinking About Your Future

Dreams and Goals

As you begin to consider your *CHOICES,* you need to think carefully about your dreams and goals. Take a few minutes and answer the following questions. (Parents, answer as you would have when you were a teen.)

1.   When I finish high school, I plan to
   - A.   Get a job at _____
   - B.   Go to college at _____
   - C.   (Other plans) _____

2.   By the time I am 25 years old I really want to be (doing what)

   _____

   _____

3.   By the time I am 25 years old I really want to be
   - A.   Living in (town) _____
   - B.   In a (type of housing) _____
   - C.   Driving a (type of vehicle) _____

4.   I would like to get married:
   - A.   Yes   No
   - B.   If yes, at what age? _____
   - C.   Describe the kind of wedding you would like.

   _____

   _____

   _____

   _____

D.   List some qualities you would want in a future spouse.

_____

_____

_____

_____

5.   If you want children, how many? _____

6.   How old do you want to be when you start your family? _____

7.   Answer the following questions:
I began this series on (date) _____

I am _____ years old and in the _____ grade.

_____ gave me this book.

My initial reaction to this book is: _____

_____

_____

_____

8.   Go to the next page and Test Your Knowledge.

Test Your Knowledge

This book is going to provide you with valuable information. Test your current knowledge with a pretest. All participating family members should take the test. The answers are provided in the back of this book and should be checked together during your Family Discussion.

Answer the following questions:

1. Can a girl become pregnant without sexual intercourse?
   A. It is impossible.
   B. It is possible but not likely.
   C. It is very possible.

2. A person can get a sexually transmitted disease without having sexual intercourse.
   A. It is impossible.
   B. It is possible but not likely.
   C. It is very possible.

3. Once a guy reaches the teenage years he produces how many sperm?
   A. About one hundred million sperm a day
   B. About one hundred million sperm a year
   C. About one hundred million sperm in a lifetime

4. A female has the most eggs for reproduction when she is
   A. Inside her mother's womb
   B. 15 years old
   C. 25 years old

5. Approximately how many sexually active teenagers get a sexually transmitted disease each year?
   A. 1 out of 2 sexually active teenagers
   B. 1 out of 4 sexually active teenagers
   C. 1 out of 10 sexually active teenagers
   D. 1 out of 20 sexually active teenagers

6. Most people with sexually transmitted diseases
    A.   Have painful sores
    B.   Have painless sores
    C.   Have sores, a rash, fever and/or pain while urinating
    D.   Have no sores or any symptoms at all

7. Which of the following sexually transmitted diseases can lead to death? (There may be more than one.)
    A.   AIDS
    B.   Gonorrhea
    C.   Human Papilloma Virus
    D.   Hepatitis B

Family Discussion

1. Students, read the questions from the first section of your Workbook entitled Dreams and Goals to your parents. Let them guess what you wrote. Put a check mark by each answer they get correct.

2. Now try to guess how your parents would have answered these same questions when they were your age. Put a check mark by each correct answer.

3. Tool #2 states that "*CHOICES* that Lead to Lifelong Success require Learning from Those with Experience." Let's hear from your parents and see how things have changed since they were teenagers. Ask your parents the following questions and learn from their experience.

    • Did your parents talk to you about sex when you were young?

    • How did you get most of your information about sex?

    • At what age did you first begin to hear about sex?

    • Did you feel your parents understood what you were experiencing as a teenager?   Explain.

    • Does this feel weird to talk about sex together as a family?

91

4.   Parents, think back to your childhood. Compare the differences in the following situations from when you were a teenager to what your children experience today.

   - Age children first began to talk about sex with their friends.

   - Age when young people first started sexual activity.

   - Number of teenagers having sex: None A few Half Most

   - Average number of sexual partners for most teenagers.

   - The age of the first girl who got pregnant in your school.

   - Pregnancy in junior high: Never Rare Some Many

   - Pregnancy in high school: Never Rare Some Many

   - Most common solution to teenage pregnancy:

        Marriage   Single Parent   Adoption   Abortion

   - Concern about sexually transmitted diseases.

   - Concern about dying from a sexually transmitted disease.

5.   Have things changed between your two generations? Explain.

6.   Are things getting better or worse?

7.   Many of today's youth get information about sex from television and movies. Parents, how much information did you get about sex from television and movies when you were growing up? Explain how things have changed.

8.   Now check your answers to the pretest.

9.   Of the questions you answered correctly on the test, were they lucky guesses or did you really know the answers? Where did you learn your information?

10.   Which answers surprised you the most?

Chapter 2
Sex: Is It Good or Bad?

Note to Parents

This chapter will briefly introduce the good and bad aspects of sex. Your child will also learn that being curious about sex and having sexual thoughts are normal and should not result in feelings of guilt. Later on in the book your child will learn the importance of bringing these thoughts under control.

In the workbook assignment, your child will be introduced to two hypothetical friends, Lori and Brian, who are about to engage in a sexual relationship. Lori has asked for your child's opinion as to whether she should go through with this or not. Your child is going to be instructed to complete a list of reasons to have sex or not to have sex. "Lori's List" will be used throughout the remainder of this series.

When you come together for your family discussion, your children may only have a few items on Lori's List. In fact, pregnancy and AIDS may be the only two reasons they have for not having sex. *DO NOT* provide any additional reasons for that side of the list. It will be better for them to discover other reasons on their own as they work through the series than for you to tell them. By the end of the series their page will be full of problems which they never considered.

Although it is important that you not give them reasons why Lori should NOT have sex, you can help your children fill out reasons why Lori and Brian may be considering sex. This might really surprise your children as you suggest reasons why teenagers have sex. Your response may help your children realize you really do understand the struggles teenagers experience. Don't overlook peer pressure, curiosity, boredom, powerful raging hormones, because it's fun and it feels good, because they want to, or because they are in love.

Another way of helping your children think about why people have sex is to ask them why people on television shows have sex. What are these people looking for? As they come up with answers they can add them to Lori's List. Don't use this as an opportunity to judge or criticize any of these shows or their characters. All you are doing right now is compiling information. If you become critical or judgmental, it may cause your children to become defensive and argumentative instead of searching for answers.

If your children are younger, they may not understand why teenagers would be interested in having sex. Remind them of the illustration used in this chapter about how their appetite has changed from milk to hamburgers and fries. Soon they will gain another normal appetite, an appetite for sex. Giving them reasons why teens are having sex will give you an opportunity to prepare them for what lies ahead.

During the family discussion you are going to be given an excellent opportunity to help your child think through some critical issues. The most common response teens have to a teenage pregnancy is, "My parents are going to kill me." This is going to be a great opportunity for you to discuss the unconditional love you have for your children.

A woman recently told me the only information she ever received from her parents about sex was one brief statement from her mother. She said she was 14-years-old when her mother looked her in the eye and simply said, "If you ever get pregnant, it will kill your father and I will kill myself." A few years later when she got pregnant, the young girl knew she had no other alternative but to have an abortion. Fear did not stop her from having sex. It did, however, prevent her from going to her parents for help when she needed them most.

Carefully think through how you are going to respond to each question during the discussion. There is nothing wrong with being honest and letting your children know you would probably be hurt and disappointed if they faced a pregnancy before marriage. But be quick to let them know these reactions have nothing to do with the love you feel for them. Your children need to know there is *nothing* they can do to make you stop loving them.

This discussion is also going to provide you with the opportunity to continue sharing your own values. Think carefully about how you would respond if your 16-year-old child or 26-year-old *single* child were involved in a pregnancy. Compare this to your response if your child was involved in a pregnancy at 26 and had been married for two years. Determine if your values about sex and pregnancy place the emphasis on marital status or the person's age.

A Tip from the Tool Box

Family Discussion time should include lots of laughter. If it starts getting too serious, try this trick. Write the following sentence on a piece of paper and have each family member read it three times as fast as possible without smiling:

**"It's silly to be silent about such a
sensational subject as sex!"**

Chapter 2

SEX: IS IT GOOD OR BAD?

Sex can be good or it can be bad. It all depends on how it is used. If you are going to make wise *CHOICES* about sex, it is important that you carefully consider all the angles. Remember,

Tool #1

CHOICES that Lead to Lifelong Success require Knowledge and Understanding

As you continue your search for SENSATIONAL SEX, you will want to figure out how to enjoy the good aspects of sex and avoid the bad.

Sex Can Be Good!

Sex Produces Babies – It is absolutely amazing that a man and woman can join their bodies in sexual intercourse and nine months later hold a precious little baby in their arms. Reproduction is incredible! But there is much more to sex than just having babies.

A Sexual Attraction is Normal – It's interesting how a six-year-old boy gets grossed out at the very thought of girls, but when he is sixteen, he can't stop thinking about them. The same thing happens for girls. The little boy who used to pull her hair and make her mad suddenly causes her heart to skip a beat. What happened? Why the change? It's simple: the boy is becoming a man and the girl is becoming a woman. Instead of repulsing each other, they are now attracted to one another.

Sexual Desires are Natural – Along with the natural attraction to each other is a natural desire for sex. Think of it this way. When you were born you had a natural appetite for milk. If someone had tried to give you a hamburger and french fries at that early age, you would have gagged and choked. But as the years went by you acquired a natural appetite to eat all kinds of food. It's the same way with sex. While sex may sound disgusting to a child, time will change that. During the teenage years a natural desire for a close relationship will develop and sex will become appealing.

Sex Can Be Fun – A sexual relationship can be fun and enjoyable. Both male and female bodies are designed to enjoy sexual intimacy. When two people really care about each other, sex can be an enjoyable way to express that love.

Sex Deepens Emotional Bonds – A sexual relationship can deepen emotional bonds and enhance a relationship. A hug may be really nice. A kiss can be very special. But two people will never be physically closer than when engaging in sexual intercourse. This intimacy can be a beautiful expression of passionate love.

Sex Can Also Cause Problems

To talk about the joys and pleasures of sex is only sharing half the truth. While it is true that sex can be very good, it can also be destructive and dangerous.

Sex Can Produce Unplanned Pregnancies – Just because a man and woman have sexual intercourse does not mean they are ready to have a baby. Although parenthood may be the last thing on their minds at the time of their passionate lovemaking, a pregnancy is always possible. An unplanned pregnancy can cause financial problems. It can interrupt an education or career path. It can also lead to serious emotional pain.

Sex Can Produce STDs – If one or both partners have had a physical relationship with another person, there is a good chance he or she could have a sexually transmitted disease without even knowing it. The disease can then be passed on to the next sexual partner. These diseases can result in a wide variety of problems ranging from painful, embarrassing sores to death. Some of these diseases can be cured; others cannot.

Sex Can Produce Emotional Scars – If sexual intercourse enhances an emotional bond, it stands to reason that if that bond is broken there can be serious emotional pain. Since a sexual relationship is not something easily forgotten, painful memories can result and haunt a person for a lifetime. Emotional scars may also produce doubts and distrust of other people. As a result future relationships can be weakened or even destroyed because of the seeds of distrust which were planted from the earlier relationship.

How To Avoid The Bad

Is it possible to have the good and avoid the bad? Yes! Sex is only destructive for those who use it recklessly. You need to realize, however, that you are growing up in a sex-saturated society. Sex is used to sell everything from cars to blue jeans. It's in movies, music, books, billboards, even the Internet. It permeates prime time television and radio. There are sex therapists, sex shops and sex hot lines. You can give it, buy it, sell it, use it, display it, abuse it and in doing so RUIN IT!

That is why the topic of sex has been selected for the training in this book. You have so many *CHOICES* to make about sex. And each *CHOICE* can lead you toward success or toward serious regrets.

Your parents have a strong desire to protect you from *DESTRUCTIVE SEX* and help you find *SENSATIONAL SEX!* You need to understand, however, that while your parents can give you guidance, the final decision will be up to you.

When you find yourself in the heat of passion, I really doubt Mom or Dad will be sitting next to you offering words of wisdom about what you should or should not be doing. At that point, it will be your responsibility to make your own *CHOICES*.

> Sex is destructive only for
> those who use it recklessly!

Warning!

Never underestimate the power of the human sex drive. Don't be surprised at the sensual thoughts and passionate desires which can flash through your mind at the most inopportune times. You may be a really good person and come from a great home. You may be a great student or athlete. But even the best of kids from the best of homes develop sexual hormones which will naturally produce sexual thoughts and desires.

The hormones raging throughout your body can leave you confused, perhaps even feeling guilty or ashamed. However, it is not "bad" or "wrong" to have sexual thoughts, and you should not feel guilty. Instead, look at each sexual thought as an opportunity to make wise *CHOICES*. With knowledge and understanding, you can find *SENSATIONAL SEX* free from guilt and hang-ups.

Respecting the Awesome Power of Sex

Consider this: If the issue were firearms instead of sex, can you imagine your mom and dad handing you the gun of your choice, patting you on the back and saying, "Have fun and enjoy yourself?"

Get real! No one in their right mind would ever hand someone a loaded gun without first teaching them to respect the awesome, yet destructive power of that firearm. In a similar manner, your parents have chosen to use this material to help you learn that sex, much like a gun, deserves tremendous respect.

Sex can be good or it can be bad. It all depends on how you use it. As you continue to expand your knowledge and understanding, you will be able to make *CHOICES* that lead to lifelong success.

At this time complete **Workbook Chapter 2** beginning on the following page.

Using Your Imagination

Think about fire.

1. List three ways that fire is good.

    A._____

    B._____

    C._____

2. List three ways that fire is bad.

    A._____

    B._____

    C._____

3. Imagine walking into your home on a cold, blustery day and seeing a big, blazing fire in the fireplace. What feelings come to your mind?

    _____

    _____

    _____

4. Now imagine walking into your home on a cold, blustery day and seeing a big, blazing fire raging out of control throughout the house. What feelings come to your mind now?

    _____

    _____

    _____

5.   Is fire good or bad? Explain.

_____

_____

_____

Now consider sex.

6.   List three reasons why sex is good.

A._____

B._____

C._____

7.   List three reasons why sex is bad.

A._____

B._____

C._____

8.   Imagine yourself at the age of 26. You've been married two years. You walk into your parent's living room and announce that you and your spouse are expecting a baby. Write the reactions you might expect from your parents and family. Be very specific.

_____

_____

_____

9.   Imagine a 16-year-old telling his or her parents that they are about to become grandparents. Write down the typical reactions you would expect from the parents.

_____

_____

_____

10.   Is sex good or is it bad? Explain.

_____

_____

_____

Consider the Problems

Let's say that Lori and Brian are two of your best friends. Lori calls and confides in you that she has decided tonight is the "big night." She is going to give up her virginity to Brian. The setting is perfect. Brian has the house to himself this weekend. No one will ever know they are there all alone. They have talked about it and decided they are both ready. Brian has had several sexual relationships and has assured Lori she won't have any regrets. He promises this will be a wonderful night they will cherish forever. It is obvious Lori is a little apprehensive and she is hoping to get your approval.

Go to Lori's List on the next page and write down all the things you think she should consider before having sex with Brian. Think of all the possible reasons why teenagers have sex and all the reasons they should consider not having sex. You will be adding additional ideas throughout the series.

Lori's List

Reasons Teens Have Sex	Reasons Not To Have Sex

Family Discussion

1. Discuss at least two ways fire can be good and two ways it can be bad. Is fire good or bad? What have you learned about fire?

2. Discuss at least two ways sex can be good and two ways it can be bad. Is sex good or bad? What have you learned about sex?

3. What are some of the primary aspects which make sex good or bad?

4. Discuss the ideas you listed on Lori's List. From the things you listed, what do you think is the main reason teens have sex? What do you think is the main reason not to have sex?

5. You were asked to write in the workbook section how typical parents might respond if their 16-year-old son or daughter told them they were about to become grandparents. Now let's see how your parents think they would feel if you announced you were involved in a teenage pregnancy. Parents, answer the following questions:

   • Would you be disappointed, hurt, and upset? Explain.

   • What do you think your first reaction would be to such an announcement?

   • If your child had been 26 and single when the pregnancy was announced, would your reaction be the same? Explain.

   • Would you want your child, whether 16 or 26, to come to you in such a situation? Explain.

Chapter 3

Super Sensational Facts on Reproduction and Fetal Development!

Note to Parents

This chapter is going to give your family incredible facts regarding human reproduction and fetal development. This should not be embarrassing. Instead, it should absolutely amaze readers of all ages. As you begin your family discussion you will be wise to set the tone of the conversation. Let your children know how fascinating this chapter was for you and how much you learned. Your positive response can help your children turn embarrassment into amazement. The discussion on fetal development will also provide you with a great opportunity to share your values regarding when life begins.

This chapter is also going to teach your children some valuable truths about how a pregnancy can occur. You will be able to emphasize this again during the discussion time. For example, a girl can get pregnant even without penetration. Although this is rare, a pregnancy can occur if a guy ejaculates near a girl's vagina. It is also possible for a girl to get pregnant when a guy withdraws before ejaculation. This is how many teenage girls get pregnant. They don't know that before ejaculation small drops of semen are released which contain hundreds of thousands of sperm.

This is the first chapter you will have the opportunity to take your discussion deeper through the Additional Discussion questions. These questions do not appear in the student book and are optional.

The information in this chapter will provide your children with tremendous knowledge which will allow them to gain a healthy respect for their body. Most of the facts came from a wonderful book called *A Child Is Born* by Nilsson. This book is filled with actual photographs of sperm, eggs, the fetus at varying stages, and childbirth. You might want to check your local bookstore or library and share it with your children. I recommend you review the book first. The pictures are graphic and leave nothing to the imagination.

A Tip from the Tool Box:

Make it a habit to have eye to eye contact with your child when you have your family discussion. This shows that you are listening and care about what your child has to say. As you show this simple common courtesy, you may find your child will quickly respond in the same manner to you.

SUPER SENSATIONAL FACTS ON REPRODUCTION AND FETAL DEVELOPMENT

As you continue your search for *SENSATIONAL SEX* it is important that you have knowledge and understanding on the facts of reproduction. But if you think reproduction is just about a sperm penetrating an egg, think again. The details of sexual reproduction are absolutely astonishing! Someone would have to be crazy if they could read the following chapter without continually saying, "Wow! That's amazing."

Just in case you think you know all about reproduction, this chapter is going to take you beyond the simple mechanics of sexual intercourse. It will provide a whole new perspective on what takes place inside your body on a daily basis.

Consider now the wonders of human reproduction!

The Male Body

In this section you will learn about the male reproductive system.

A boy usually begins sexual maturity around 12 to 13 years of age. At this time the male sex hormone, **testosterone**, causes numerous changes. Growth spurts will cause boys to finally grow taller than most girls. Their voices begin to change. They develop hair on their face and body and their muscles become larger.

It is also during this time that a boy starts to produce **sperm** from his **testicles**. The testicles are attached to the body by a pouch of skin called the **scrotum**. To produce sperm normally, the testicles must be cooler than the rest of the body. Therefore, the scrotum is suspended away from the body to provide this lower temperature. The scrotum stays at 95° F or 35° C.[1] Think about it. If the scrotum was not suspended from the body, reproduction would be impossible!

A healthy young male will produce about **100,000,000 (one hundred million) sperm each day**. That's more than **one thousand sperm a second**.[2] Wow! Is that amazing or what?

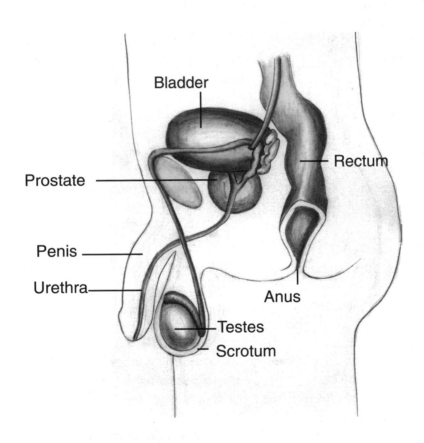

The Male Reproductive System

Each sperm is so small that it can only be seen through a microscope. A sperm consists of a head and a tail. Within the head of each sperm is a selection of the father's genetic material to create a new, unique person. The sperm wiggles its tail back and forth, swimming with only one goal: to fertilize an egg. In this drawing, you can see the head and tail.

Sperm leaves the male body through a small tube inside the **penis** called the **urethra**. This is the same tube used to eliminate urine from a man's body. Sperm leaves the body in a milky looking fluid called semen. When the sperm leaves the male body, this is called **ejaculation**. Each ejaculation produces about one-half to one teaspoon of semen. That may not sound like much, but it contains up to **500 million sperm** all striving to win the race to the female's egg.[3]

A man may ejaculate as a result of sexual excitement. He may also ejaculate during his sleep. Ejaculation during sleep is called **nocturnal emission** or a **wet dream**. This is normal and is caused by certain reflexes triggered during sleep.

The Female Body

In this section you will learn about the female reproductive system.

Girls typically begin sexual maturity around 11 to 12 years of age. During this time there will be a growth spurt. Estrogen, the female sex hormone, will cause the breasts to begin forming and hips to widen. Bodily hair will begin to grow, soon followed by menstruation and ovulation. At this time a girl will have the ability to have a baby.

The **uterus**, or womb, is located inside the lower abdomen of the female. This muscular organ resembles the shape and size of a small pear, but it is capable of growing much larger when a woman is pregnant. When a girl reaches the age of 11 to 14, her uterus will prepare for nurturing a fertilized egg. Every month the uterus will build a rich lining where the baby can grow for nine months. However, if the egg is not fertilized by a male sperm, the lining in the uterus is not needed and is discarded. This process is called **menstruation, menstrual cycle or monthly period**. This cycle occurs about every 28 days.

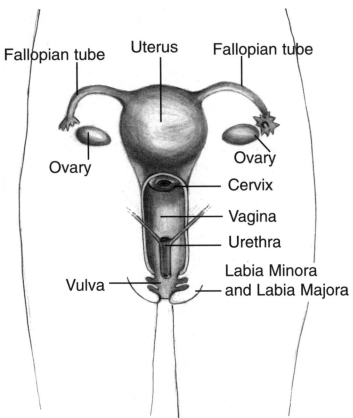

The Female Reproductive System

As the lining of the uterus is discarded, the woman experiences a bloody discharge from her vagina for three to seven days. The **vagina** is a special opening between a woman's legs. It is also referred to as the birth canal, because this is where a baby passes at birth. When a woman experiences her menstrual cycle, she can use a variety of different products to keep her clothes from becoming soiled.

Once the lining of the uterus has been discarded, the process will start all over and continue every month. A woman will menstruate about 400 times during her life. Then typically when she is in her late 40's or early 50's, her monthly menstrual cycle will stop. This is called **menopause**. At this time she will no longer be fertile (capable of having a baby) and can no longer become pregnant.

The other important event which takes place each month inside the female body is called **ovulation**. During ovulation, one or both **ovaries** release a ripened egg (also called ovum) into the **fallopian tube**. Each egg contains the mother's genetic material necessary to produce a new life.

Women do not continue to produce new eggs. Unlike men, who produce sperm on a daily basis, women are born with eggs in their ovaries. In fact, a female has the most eggs when she is still inside her mother's womb. By the fifth month of pregnancy, **an unborn baby girl will have about five million eggs in her ovaries**. At birth the number will have dropped to about **one or two million**. By the early teenage years, she will have about **300,000** eggs. Of course, she will only need about 400 eggs since she will only **ovulate about 400 times during her life**.[4] By the time a woman reaches menopause, there are no healthy eggs left in her ovaries and she is no longer capable of having a baby.

Ovulation occurs about **14 days** before the woman's next menstrual cycle. Once the egg is released, she will be fertile, or capable of becoming pregnant, for approximately 24 hours. Some adult women are able to tell fairly accurately when they are ovulating. They often have a small discharge, slight cramping sensation, and even a slight change in their body temperature. If a woman wants to get pregnant, she needs to have sexual intercourse at the time of ovulation or during the three to five days before ovulation.

Teenage girls and many women often have irregular cycles and are unable to tell when they are fertile. *Because of this unpredictable cycle and not knowing exactly when she might ovulate, a girl needs to realize she might become pregnant almost any time she has sexual intercourse.*

When the egg is released from the ovary, it travels down the **fallopian tube**. It is inside this small, delicate tube where fertilization takes place. The egg must be fertilized by the sperm within **24 hours** or the egg will disintegrate.[5] Remember, a woman is only fertile when she ovulates. Usually, this is also when she is most easily aroused sexually.

Sexual Intercourse

When a man and woman are sexually aroused their bodies prepare for sexual intercourse. Normally, the man's penis is soft. However, when he becomes sexually aroused his penis becomes erect or stiff. An **erection** is the result of blood filling the inside of the penis. (The blood does not come out. It stays inside the penis.) Once the penis is erect it can be inserted into the woman's vagina. When a woman becomes sexually aroused her body produces vaginal secretions which make it easier to insert the penis.

When a man ejaculates during sexual intercourse millions of sperm travel out his penis and are deposited inside the woman's vagina. At that moment the race is on as the eager sperm begin the six to seven inch journey toward the fallopian tubes in search of an egg.

The woman's moist mucus secretions allow the sperm to live for three to five days as they search for an egg. Therefore, if two people have sex on a Friday night and she ovulates the next Monday, the eager sperm can still be swimming around the fallopian tubes searching for the egg.

If a man removes his penis before he ejaculates (called "withdrawal"), the woman can still get pregnant. Even before ejaculation, small drops of seminal fluid are released from the penis. These small drops contain thousands of sperm which can still cause a pregnancy.

If a man ejaculates near the opening of a woman's vagina, but not inside her vagina, there is still a chance she could become pregnant. Therefore, it is possible for a pregnancy to occur without sexual intercourse, but this would be rare. Never underestimate the determination of the sperm to find the female's egg! Remember, it only takes one sperm to fertilize an egg.

Conception

The following drawing shows a sperm penetrating an egg.

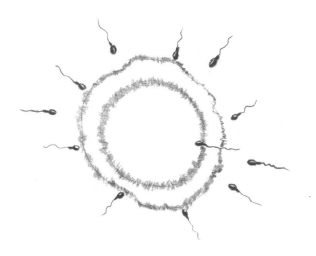

Conception occurs when the head of the sperm penetrates the egg. This usually takes place in the upper one-third of the fallopian tube. The chemical composition of the egg immediately changes, making it impossible for any other sperm to penetrate the egg.

Although the egg is smaller than a grain of salt, it is far larger than the sperm. When the sperm penetrates the egg, the sperm and egg become one cell. This single tiny cell holds hereditary material passed down from generation to generation from both the father and mother.

Once inside the egg, the sperm releases the father's genetic material. His 23 chromosomes are joined with the mother's 23 chromosomes. Instantly the child's sex, height, facial features, blood type, skin, hair and eye color, and other features are determined.

The father's chromosome determines whether the baby will be a boy or girl. Some sperm have a Y chromosome producing a boy and some have an X chromosome producing a girl.

Within **12 hours** after conception the tiny single cell divides into two cells. This division continues every 12 to 15 hours. The fertilized egg remains in the fallopian tube for about three days before it enters the uterus. About five to eight days after conception, **the egg will plant itself inside the rich uterine lining**. This process prevents the woman from having her next monthly menstrual cycle, which is often a woman's first indication that she may be pregnant.[6]

Multiple Births

Multiple births can occur in two different ways. **Fraternal twins** develop when more than one egg is released. If both eggs are fertilized, fraternal twins will occur. (If three eggs are released and fertilized, triplets will occur, and so on.) Although these babies will share the same birthday, they will be no more alike than any other brother or sister. One of the twins might be a boy, the other a girl. One might be very tall with blond hair, the other short with brown hair.

Identical twins are produced when a fertilized egg splits for unknown reasons and develops into two individuals. In this case both eggs will have identical genes. The two individuals will be the same sex and look alike.

Miscarriage, Stillbirth and Abortion

A **miscarriage** is the unintentional termination of a pregnancy before the twentieth week. A miscarriage may occur for a variety of reasons, but in most cases something went wrong with the chromosomes, such as having too many or too few.

After the twentieth week, an accidental termination is called a **stillbirth**. When a woman chooses to terminate a pregnancy, it is called an **abortion**.

The Differences in Males and Females

- Starting at age 12 to 14 a boy's body produces sperm every day. A girl is born with all her eggs and will never produce any more.

- Once a young man reaches sexual maturity in his early teens he will be *fertile* for the rest of his life. A woman is *infertile* most of her life. She is fertile for only about 24 hours each month. Most girls and many women do not know exactly when they are fertile.

- Teenage boys, as well as adult men, are capable of producing a baby every time they engage in sexual intercourse. In fact, men over age 80 have fathered babies. A woman will stop being fertile around the age of 50. After that time she will not be able to have a baby.

Sensational Facts on Fetal Development!

If the facts about reproduction amazed you, take a look at the facts on fetal development. You don't remember, but you experienced this inside your mother. Notice how fast the development takes place!

- **Day 1** – Conception occurs and the journey to the uterus begins.
- **Days 5 to 8** –The fertilized egg implants in the upper portion of the uterus. Although it has expanded to 200 cells, it is no larger than a grain of sand.
- **Days 10 to 14** – The mother misses her first menstrual period.
- **Day 21** – The heart begins to beat.
- **4 Weeks** – The **embryo** is about 1/4 inch long. The brain and backbone are forming, while the heart begins to pump blood to the liver and into the aorta.
- **5 to 6 Weeks** – The embryo is just over a half inch long. The skeleton is complete and the eyes, nose, and mouth have formed. The arms and legs are very short at this stage, but ten little fingers are now developing.

- **8 Weeks** – Every organ is now in place and functioning! The embryo is now called a fetus which is Latin for "young one." The fetus has the definite appearance of a baby even though it is only about one-and-a-half inches long and weighs less than a half-ounce.

8 Week Fetus

- **10 to 12 Weeks** –The fetus, now 3 inches long, can exercise its tiny arms and legs. It sleeps, awakens, sucks its thumb, gets the hiccups and urinates. Facial expressions begin as the fetus can squint, frown, and open and close its mouth.
- **4 Months** – The fetus is now about 4 inches long. It actively kicks, swims and turns somersaults, but the mother cannot feel the activity – yet. The arms are now long enough for the hands to grasp each other and fingernails begin to appear. The eyes have now closed and will not open again until 7 months. It is now obvious if the fetus is a boy or girl. The mother's abdomen is beginning to swell.
- **5 Months** –The pregnancy is halfway over. Although the fetus has been actively moving for several weeks, the mother just now begins to feel the movements. The outer ear is fully formed and the fetus responds to sound, especially loud noise. The fetus now has colored hair on its head and eyebrows.
- **6 Months** – The baby now weighs over 1 pound and has a chance of survival if born at this point.

- **7 Months** – The baby now weighs over 2 pounds and will begin to put on about half a pound a week. The fetus can now recognize voices.
- **8 Months** – The delicate skin begins to thicken as the fetus continues to put on weight. The baby is now about 18 inches long and weighs almost 4 pounds.
- **9 Months** – The time is finally here! The baby will be ready for delivery by the end of this month. The average baby weighs 7 pounds and is 20 inches long. It's been about 36 to 40 weeks since the sperm penetrated the egg and now it's time for the baby to enter the world.[7]

**Baby in the womb
at 9 months**

Labor and Delivery

The birth of a baby begins when the mother experiences consecutive contractions called **labor pains**. These usually last about 6 to 20 hours (less if she has given birth before.) During labor the baby's head pushes downward into the **birth canal** or vagina. The **cervix** (the opening of the uterus) gradually opens until it is fully dilated to about 10 cm (about 4 inches.) The baby then passes through the birth canal and out the vaginal opening.

If the baby's bottom is pushing down into the birth canal instead of its head, it is called a **breech birth**. This makes the birth process more complicated, and the doctor may choose to perform a **cesarean section** in which the baby is delivered through an incision in the mother's abdomen.[8]

As the baby enters the world, the first breath of air is taken and the parents will hear the marvelous sound of their baby's first cry.

The Amazing Truth!

Sexual reproduction and fetal development are absolutely amazing! Reproduction is far more than a sperm penetrating an egg. Fetal development is much more than simple cell division. Whether or not you plan to become a father or mother anytime soon, your body is continuously working in preparation for that special day.

At this time complete **Workbook Chapter 3** beginning on the following page.

Test Your Knowledge

1. Fill in the Blank
   A. A healthy male will produce about how many sperm per second?

   _____

   B. Each time a male ejaculates there are approximately _____ sperm trying to do what?

   _____

   C. Why is it important for the scrotum to be suspended from the man's body?

   _____

   D. Most women will have a menstrual cycle and ovulate about how many times in their life?

   _____

   E. How much time does the egg have to be fertilized before it disintegrates?

   _____

   F. Is it the male's sperm or the female's egg which determines if a baby is a girl or boy?

   _____

   G. On which day of fetal development does the fertilized egg implant in the uterus?

   _____

   H. The heart begins to beat on what day?

   _____

I. Fetus is a Latin word which means what?

_____

J. By which week of fetal development is every organ in place and functioning?

_____

K. If the baby is born at _____ months, it has a chance of survival.

L. After about _____ weeks the baby is ready for birth.

2. <u>True or False</u>

A. There is a chance a girl can become pregnant almost any time she has sexual intercourse. True   False

B. Sperm have several purposes.   True   False

C. A woman tends to be sexually aroused more easily when she is most fertile.   True   False

D. A man could become a father even into his eighties.   True   False

E. A woman always knows when she is fertile.   True   False

F. A woman can become pregnant even if there is no penetration by the penis.   True   False

G. A man will produce about 100,000,000 sperm in his lifetime.   True   False

H. A woman has the most eggs for reproduction when she is 16 years old.   True   False

I. A man is capable of producing a baby every time he has sexual intercourse.   True   False

3.   List three amazing facts described in this chapter.

A._____

B._____

C._____

4.   Go back to Lori's List. Is there anything you should explain to her about reproduction?

Family Discussion

1.   Check your answers in the back of this book.

2.   As a family, describe several amazing facts discussed in this chapter regarding males.

3.   Now describe several amazing facts regarding females.

4.   What amazed you most about fetal development?

5.   What in your opinion is the most amazing fact of all?

6.   What were some of the significant differences between men and women which were discussed in this chapter?

7.   Why are the following statements significant in terms of a possible pregnancy?

- A male is fertile every time he has sex.

- Although it is rare, it is possible for a woman to become pregnant without penetration.

- Even if a man withdraws his penis during sexual intercourse before he ejaculates, small drops of semen have usually been released.

(Additional Discussion Questions are on the next page.)

Additional Discussion

Note: These questions are optional. They do not appear in the student book. If you want to take your discussion further you can continue with these questions.

⇒ Ask your children if they have any questions about what they read on reproduction.

⇒ At conception, you received 23 chromosomes from your mother and 23 from your father. Take your shoes off and compare toes. Did you get your toes from your mother or father? Now compare your thumbs. What about your eyes, nose, height, and hair color?

⇒ Parents, tell your children what it was like when you were expecting them. How did mom feel physically? How big did she get? How much weight did she gain? Who drove her to the hospital? How long was her labor? How much did the baby weigh? How did she feel the first time she held her baby?

⇒ If you adopted your child, you may not have all the answers, but you can share what you do know. How did you feel when you got word you were going to get a baby? How long had you waited for this wonderful event? How much did your baby weigh? How did you feel the first time you held your baby?

⇒ Take this opportunity to teach your child *your* values regarding when life begins and when that life has value. At conception? When the heart beats and brain waves are present? At birth? Explain why you hold these values.

Note: The next chapter, "I Had a Dream," is my personal story. You might want to consider sitting down as a family and listening to the tape or CD together as I tell you first hand about the *CHOICES* I made in my life. (See the back of this book for information on ordering tapes or CDs.)

References

[1]Lennart Nilsson, M.D., *A Child is Born*, Delacorte Press, New York, NY, 1990; 26.
[2]Ibid.
[3]Ibid., 29.
[4]Ibid., 17-21.
[5]Ibid.
[6]Ibid., 57-66.
[7]Ibid., 75-147.
[8]Ibid., 41-149.

BOOK TWO

SECTION TWO

WOW! IT COULD HAPPEN TO ME!

Now that you know how amazing reproduction and fetal development are, it's time to learn some of the problems that can be associated with sex. As you continue in your search for *SENSATIONAL SEX,* you need to understand the possible dangers and how to avoid them.

> What you don't know can
> really hurt you!

Note to Parents

In this chapter I will share my story with your family. I will also reveal to your children that I promote the concept of sexual abstinence until marriage. After you read my story, you will understand why I have devoted my life to working with today's youth.

Pay close attention to the various details given in this story. You will be able to refer back to my situation in future family discussions.

A Tip from the Tool Box:

A government study indicated that the pregnancy rate is lower among young people who have a greater number of shared activities with their parents.[1] Go places with your child. Do fun things together. Dream with your child about all the exciting possibilities of life.

---

[1] Resnick, Michael, D., Ph.D., et al., "Protecting Adolescents from Harm: Findings from the National Longitudinal Study on Adolescent Health," *Journal of the American Medical Association,* 9/10/97.

Chapter 4

I HAD A DREAM!

Throughout the rest of this book you will read true stories about people whose lives have been changed, for better or worse, because of the *CHOICES* they made about sex. I'll start by telling you my own story. After reading it, you will understand why I am devoting my life to talking with teenagers about sex.

I was born in Lubbock, Texas in 1951. Lubbock's greatest claim to fame was rock 'n' roll star Buddy Holly. By age twelve I too had aspirations of being a celebrity, making my entire family and community proud of my accomplishments.

My father managed grain elevators. Mom was a school teacher. I had an older brother and sister who, from my point of view, were perfect, popular, "A" students who constantly received all kinds of awards and honors. I, on the other hand, was not an "A" student and had received no awards or honors. But I had a secret dream that would someday change everything.

We were the typical family of the '50s and '60s. We always ate breakfast and dinner together at the kitchen table. Every Sunday we went to church. Mom and Dad were both Sunday School teachers, scout leaders and active members of the PTA.

The Dream

My early childhood consisted of school, piano lessons, church, and girl scouts. Once I reached seventh grade, I dropped scouts for tennis. That, you see, was my secret dream. I was determined to become a professional tennis player.

I started entering city tournaments in the seventh grade. The next year I collected my first trophies. My first big break came in the ninth grade when the high school tennis coach saw me play and invited me to work out each day with the high school team. At that time, ninth grade was still in junior high. For a ninth grader to practice with the high school team every day was a dream come true! Even better, the coach entered me in several out-of-town tournaments that year with the varsity team. This was just the break I needed to achieve my secret dream.

As a sophomore I continued to live and breathe tennis. Not content to simply be on the tennis team, I was determined to make the varsity team and compete in all the out-of-town tournaments. That was tough, fighting to hold my position week after week. But when the season ended that year, I had accomplished my goal. I was the only sophomore who made it to every tournament. I didn't win any, but there was always next year to bring home the trophies.

Romance

Tennis was not the only highlight of my sophomore year. Just before traveling season started, I had a blind date. Chuck was a year ahead of me in school, a straight "A" student and a member of the student council. At 6'4" and 220 pounds he was, naturally, a football player. The best thing about this guy: he liked me. He was my first serious boyfriend.

From the first night we met Chuck and I were inseparable, having a date every Friday, Saturday, and Sunday evening. Each date would begin by going to a party, the show, or dinner. But each always ended at our special place where we could be all alone. There was nothing I liked more than Chuck holding me in his arms and passionately kissing me. I thought if I died right there in his arms I would die the happiest sixteen year old on the face of the earth! Oh sure, the kissing would get pretty hot and heavy at times, but what could it hurt? We were just kissing and kissing never hurt anything!

Everyone Does It

One of my best friends was a girl a few years older than me. I looked up to her and enjoyed our heart-to-heart talks. One day, when we were having one of our talks, she asked me very directly, "Marilyn, are you and Chuck having sex?"

"No, we aren't," I replied. "We're kind of struggling with this, but we have promised each other we are going to wait until we get married." She started laughing. At first I wasn't sure what I had said that was so funny. Then I realized she was laughing at the concept of waiting until marriage.

She stopped laughing and got very serious. She looked me straight in the eye and said, "Marilyn, sex is no big deal. Everyone does it. And I assure you, no one waits until marriage." Then she gave me a list of all her friends who were having sex. "It's not hurting them," she said. "And I assure you, it won't hurt you and Chuck."

Something about that conversation really bothered me. I told Chuck about it that evening. We both agreed that it didn't matter what everyone else was doing. We were not going to have sex until we got married. Although there was a great deal of passion between us, we were convinced we could control the physical side of our relationship.

Playing with Fire

If you have ever sat around a campfire and watched the fire burn out, you know there are two options: you can let it die or you can add more wood. Chuck and I found ourselves in a similar situation. After awhile, kissing wasn't all that special anymore. The fire between us was growing cold. We were left with two *CHOICES*: we could walk away from our fading relationship or we could add a little more fuel to the fire. We quickly learned that by just a little touching the passion was rekindled. It was like a game – a fun, exciting game. What could it hurt? After all, we were in control and could stop anytime.

I often thought about what my friend said: "*Everyone* is having sex." That still didn't matter. There was no way we were going to go all the way. After all, there is a big difference between a little touching and having sex.

133

A New Dream

Our relationship continued through the next year. Chuck was now a senior and I was a junior. We began to talk about marriage. Chuck occasionally mentioned it, but I became consumed with the idea! I had it all figured out. I would get my engagement ring for Valentine's Day my senior year. We would be married a few weeks after I graduated. I could hardly wait to walk down the aisle as a beautiful bride in a gorgeous white gown in a church full of friends and family.

As the dream of my wedding became bigger than life, my secret dream of becoming a professional tennis player began to fade. Although I made the varsity team and again went to every tournament, my drive and determination were gone. My goal of bringing home trophies had been replaced with a passion for romance.

Fire Out of Control

The game Chuck and I had started playing the year before was now all consuming. Just as the kissing did not satisfy for long, touching soon lost its excitement. We found we needed a little more to satisfy. And then one night it happened. We didn't plan it. It just happened. We went all the way.

When I got home that night, I stared at myself in the mirror. It was strange. I didn't look any different, but I felt different – not like I expected though. I thought a person was supposed to feel joy and excitement after having sex, but I felt cheap and disappointed. All this time I thought we controlled the game, but now I realized the game had controlled us from the very beginning.

As the weeks and months went by, I was surprised at the effect sex had on our relationship. I thought it was supposed to bring a couple closer together. It didn't. Now that we had gone all the way, there was nothing new to make the relationship more exciting. As Chuck's senior year ended, we seemed to spend most of our time arguing.

My senior year brought more difficult changes. Chuck was now in college and heavily pursued by a fraternity. His life was now filled with parties, meetings, study groups – and little time for me. It was clear that our relationship was coming to an end.

The Shock

The pain was so deep. How do you walk away from your first love? How do you leave someone you have been with for two years? Someone to whom you had given *everything*?

Although we continued to date during the fall, I decided I should refocus on my first love, tennis. I had lost momentum my junior year and had probably destroyed any hopes of a scholarship. But maybe with enough work, I could still make a college team. I could pour myself once more into tennis and still graduate as someone special.

But then, in November, the unthinkable happened. I realized I was pregnant. "NO! . . . This could not be happening!"

For two weeks Chuck and I screamed and yelled at each other as we tried to sort through this nightmare. We were good kids, from good homes. This just didn't happen in families like ours. We were scared and felt very alone. I was 17, he was 18. These were supposed to be the carefree years of our lives, but suddenly we were thrust into a very adult situation.

Back in the late '60s there were only two viable options to a teenage pregnancy: marriage or adoption. We never discussed adoption. Chuck may have wished he could have escaped that easily, but he knew he had to do the "right thing." Any respectable young man who got a girl pregnant back then knew he would have to marry her.

Chuck wasn't happy about the situation. He was a very intelligent young man and was sure this would destroy his future. He was convinced of three things: (1) his parents were going to kill him; (2) he would never finish college; and (3) he would have to sell his car. To an eighteen-year-old guy, a car was the greatest possession on earth. Chuck had worked long and hard for that car and now he was sure he would have to sell it.

Spreading the Pain Around

It was a Sunday afternoon when Chuck finally got the courage to tell his parents I was pregnant — one of the hardest things he ever did. Chuck had a great deal of respect and love for his parents and didn't want to hurt them. He was afraid they would tell him to pack his bags and get out of the house.

He braced himself for their response. To his surprise they simply said, "We knew something was wrong by the way you've been acting lately. What do you plan to do, and how can we help?" He was amazed at their response. Then he explained that we had decided to get married the following weekend, if my parents would sign the marriage papers and not kill him!

Next, Chuck had to face my mother and father and tell them I was pregnant. Not an easy task, but he knew it was his responsibility. Chuck was surprised when his dad volunteered to go along for support. He said his father cried all the way over to my house and kept saying, "I'm sorry, son; we should have talked about this sooner." Chuck learned so much about his parents that day and the love they had for him.

Chuck and his father had barely walked through our front door when Chuck announced to my parents, "Marilyn's pregnant and we want to get married." My mother began crying hysterically and ran out of the room. My dad, on the other hand, was very calm and told Chuck that he felt everyone needed a little time to think this over. He suggested we all get together in a few days.

As Chuck and his father walked out the door, Daddy did something I will never forget. He walked over to me, wrapped his arms around me, hugged me, and gently said, "It's okay. We will all work this out together." Never in my life had I broken my father's heart more than at that very moment. And yet, never in my life did I feel my father's love more.

Our Families Meet

Two days later both families met. I had no idea what was about to take place. With a firm voice and great conviction Daddy turned to Chuck and said, "I appreciate the fact that you're willing to marry my daughter. But I need to know if you really believe you're capable of caring for a wife and baby. If you don't feel you're ready for this, we will walk out right now, release you of all responsibilities and handle this our own way."

Everything inside me was screaming, "What do you mean we will handle this our own way? What is our own way? What are you talking about? He wants to marry me. Don't talk him out of this!" But I knew I had to be silent. I had already done enough damage and hurt enough people.

Daddy continued, "However, if you decide to marry Marilyn, I expect you to take care of both my daughter and this baby. Now, do you really believe at 18 years of age you are capable of doing this?"

The silence in the room was deafening! My heart was pounding. It seemed like an eternity before Chuck finally looked away from my father and looked directly at me. He slowly said, "I love Marilyn and I want to marry her. I will take care of her and the baby."

My Wedding

Four days later, on a Saturday evening, November 30, 1968, I walked down the aisle of the church at my wedding. There was total silence as Daddy escorted me toward the front where Chuck and the minister stood.

I had always dreamed of wearing a gorgeous white gown at my wedding. But when Mom handed me the credit card the day before the wedding and painfully said, "I guess you should go buy something to wear," I didn't know what was appropriate. What does a seventeen-year-old bride, six weeks pregnant, wear? With great disappointment I selected a pink, street length linen dress.

Daddy and I made our way down the aisle, passing all the empty pews. Only my mother, brother and sister sat on the left side of the church, while Chuck's family sat on the first row on the right. The minister spoke briefly and within a few minutes it was all over. I was now Mrs. Charles Morris.

This was nothing like the elaborate wedding I had so carefully planned in my mind. Who would have ever guessed the game we began playing would have led to this? For the first time I began to understand that the *CHOICES* we make in life have consequences. But my consequences didn't stop at the wedding.

Reality Sets In

It was strange waking up the next morning in our little one room apartment. It took me a moment to figure out where I was. But nausea suddenly brought me to my senses. Bolting out of bed, I ran to the bathroom. I remember thinking, what an attractive way to start your marriage, listening to your wife throw up her guts. This was something Chuck was going to have to get used to though. The morning sickness lasted several more weeks.

Facing Disappointment

Monday morning I had to face the world. I went directly to the school office to announce that I was married. Although this was an unusual situation, school policy did state that married students could remain in school. The school counselor was quick to remind me, however, that married students could not participate in extracurricular activities. What did it really matter? The thought of wearing a maternity dress to the senior prom was not exactly enticing!

I was given a form for each teacher, instructing them to change my name on their records. I knew I had to see one teacher first before word spread that I was married. I went directly to his class and asked if I could talk with him in the hall. This wasn't just any teacher; this was my tennis coach.

My voice shook as I said, "There's something I need to tell you. Chuck and I got married Saturday night." At first he thought I was kidding. But when I lifted my left hand and showed him my ring, he knew this was for real.

His shocked expression was becoming all too familiar. With a sigh he simply said, "You know what this means, don't you?"

"Yes. I'm sorry, Coach." While giving up the senior prom wasn't that hard, giving up tennis was another story.

Word quickly spread that I was married. By the time I got to the last period of the day, everyone on the tennis team had already heard the news. As I entered the dressing room, all the girls quickly gathered to see my ring. But moments later they hurried out to the courts. I was left standing all alone gazing at this room that held so many memories. I opened my locker, gathered my clothes and tennis racket, looked around the room one last time and walked out the door.

As I walked away from the tennis courts, I knew my secret childhood dream had come to an end once and for all.

Graduation

I did graduate that spring along with my 700 classmates. And just as I had once envisioned, people did take note as I walked across the stage. But instead of whispering to each other, "She's the tennis player," they were saying, "She's the pregnant girl."

More than Just Me

It's strange. When I chose to become sexually involved, I thought it was just about me. After all, it was a game I chose to play. It was *my* virginity and *my* reputation on the line. Later I began to realize how self-centered I had been.

This wasn't just about *me*, *my* dreams and *my* goals. It was also about Chuck and *his* dreams and goals. But it didn't stop there either. It was also about our parents, extended families, friends, and most of all, it was about a little baby girl who was born one month after I graduated from high school.

Today

Many years have now gone by. And yes, Chuck and I are still married – for 31 years in fact. Our little baby girl is now a 30-year-old woman, a wife and a mother. We also have another married daughter who is 27. These two young ladies are absolutely the joy of our lives!

No, I never did become a professional tennis player. I did split sets, however, with a retired pro in the finals of a city tournament when I was 25, but I never got any further than that.

As for Chuck's three greatest fears: Obviously, his parents did not kill him. Instead, they actually became a great support and encouragement to us in those early years of marriage. And yes, he did finish college. It took five years of hard work, but he did it. And no, he didn't have to sell his car. In fact, we had that car for six more years.

So what do we do now? Chuck and I run an educational organization called Aim for Success which has challenged hundreds of thousands of teenagers throughout the country to think about their life, dreams and goals. Chuck runs the company and I speak and oversee the various programs.

Paying the Price

Perhaps you are thinking, "Well, everything turned out all right for you after all." If by *everything* you mean:

- Sacrificing my dreams of tennis, college, and a beautiful wedding.
- Preventing our relationship from growing in a healthy way because of premarital sex.
- Forcing us to grow up overnight while all our friends were enjoying their youth.
- Causing humiliation and disappointment for our parents.
- Causing much pain and embarrassment for both me and Chuck.

Yes, I guess *everything* has turned out all right for us, but what a price we had to pay as we endured pain and hard work through the years to make it turn out.

Taking a Stand: Condoms or Abstinence?

In the beginning of the book, I told you I would tell you whether I promote the use of condoms or abstinence. Well, here's my answer.

Chuck and I never used condoms, pills, or any other form of birth control device to prevent a pregnancy. But let's change the story for a moment. Let's say we did use a condom and it did protect me from the pregnancy. No doubt I would have graduated from high school and gone on to college and perhaps pursued my dream of tennis. What a difference a condom would have made!

Of course, all of these dreams and goals would have been fulfilled without Chuck because we were about to break up when I got pregnant. But there would have been other boys to take Chuck's place. With each new boyfriend the game would have started all over: a little kissing, a little touching and after sex there's nothing new left to do.

So I would have gone to the *next* boyfriend and the game would have started again: a little kissing, a little touching and after sex there's nothing new left to do. I believe my life would have become a total disaster as I searched in vain for a meaningful relationship.

Do I wish Chuck and I had practiced safe sex by using a condom? No! I wish we had truly been committed to sexual abstinence until marriage. We learned that anyone can say they are committed to abstinence, but it takes *knowledge and understanding* to make the *CHOICE* for sexual abstinence. Chuck and I did not have the *knowledge, understanding or strong commitment* required to achieve sexual abstinence until marriage.

I am convinced that if we had truly been committed to abstinence we would have developed an incredible friendship. We would have had a blast together throughout high school without ever jeopardizing each other's dreams and goals.

Would we be married today? Who knows. I do know that today Chuck is my very best friend, but it took years of hard work to get to this point. What a difference it would have made if we had focused on developing a deep friendship while dating and had fun developing the sexual side after we were married.

What about You?

As you continue to search for the secret of *SENSATIONAL SEX* let me encourage you to:

- Never underestimate the power of the sex drive.

- Realize the slightest amount of physical activity, which usually begins with passionate kissing, can become an addictive game. Once you get started, you constantly need a little more to satisfy.

- Realize a *healthy* relationship with another person should never destroy your dreams and goals. It should, however, help you fulfill your dreams and goals.

- Realize the importance of sharing your dreams and goals with others. Allow your parents and other caring adults to dream with you and encourage you.

Remember, the *CHOICES* you make about sex can lead to lifelong success or a lifetime of regret.

At this time complete **Workbook Chapter 4** beginning on the following page.

Reading Between the Lines

1. Go back to the section in this chapter called "Playing with Fire." What was holding Chuck and Marilyn's relationship together?

    _____

    _____

    _____

2. Is that a healthy foundation for a relationship? Why or Why not?

    _____

    _____

    _____

3. What is peer pressure?

    _____

    _____

4. Describe below the peer pressure Marilyn faced and how she responded to it.

    _____

    _____

    _____

5. Describe below the peer pressure you see today in:

    school – _____

    television –_____

    movies –_____

    music –_____

    other –_____

6. Marilyn could have had it all. She could have graduated from high school, gone off to college, continued her dream of playing tennis, found romance, gotten married, and had a family. Unfortunately, Marilyn didn't have enough knowledge and understanding about life and relationships to make wise *CHOICES*. Write down the *CHOICES* Marilyn could have made which would have allowed her to have it all.

    _____

    _____

    _____

    _____

7. Go back to Lori's List in Workbook Chapter 2. Are there things you can add to the list?

8. Now that you have read Marilyn's story, go to the next page and write out what you hope will be your story. Include your dreams and goals for the future. What's going to happen after high school? What career path do you want to take? What type of people will you date? If you plan to marry, include your marriage and wedding plans. Describe the person you would want to marry. What about children? Do you see a family in the future? If so, when?

My Story

_____

_____

_____

_____

_____

_____

_____

_____

_____

_____

_____

_____

_____

_____

_____

_____

_____

_____

_____

_____

_____

_____

_____

_____

_____

Family Discussion

1.   In the section entitled "Romance," Marilyn stated: "Oh sure, the kissing would get pretty hot and heavy at times, but what could it hurt? We were just kissing, and kissing never hurt anything!" Is that true? Can passionate kissing be dangerous? Explain.

2.   Marilyn's friend told her, "Sex is no big deal. Everyone does it. And I assure you, no one waits until marriage." How many lies can you count in that statement? What is the truth in each case?

3.   Did sex bring Chuck and Marilyn closer?

4.   The *CHOICES* Marilyn made about sex changed her life forever. Although good things eventually came from her story, she faced many disappointments. Discuss the outcome of the following situations:

- her first sexual experience
- her senior prom
- her wedding
- her graduation
- her tennis career

5.   Would contraceptives have improved the outcome of Marilyn's life?

Additional Discussion

⇒ Discuss how you answered question 6 in your Workbook.

⇒ Marilyn said she learned that having sex was not just about one person. What did she mean? How many people were affected by her decision to have sex?

⇒ Ask your children if they would like to share the story they wrote entitled "My Story."

Note to Parents

The discussion in this chapter can provide another occasion for a wonderful heart to heart talk. While your children are probably familiar with the options of an unplanned teenage pregnancy, the true stories might help them to see that there are no easy solutions.

You will also be given another opportunity to share your unconditional love for your children while stating your values about sex and pregnancy and your views on abortion.

A Tip from the Tool Box:

Spend time with your children. It's difficult to build a close relationship if you aren't spending time together. Although parents now spend 10 to 12 hours a week less with their children than parents of the 1960s, they are making a difference by being home at key times of the day – morning, after school, dinner, and bedtime.[1]

---

[1] Resnick, Michael, D., Ph.D., et al., "Protecting Adolescents from Harm: Findings from the National Longitudinal Study on Adolescent Health," *Journal of the American Medical Association,* 9/10/97.

Chapter 5

PREGNANCY

Facts

- About 1 million teenage girls get pregnant each year. That's about 1 out of 5 sexually active girls.[1]
- Pregnancy is the top reason why teenage girls are hospitalized.[2]
- 7 out of 10 adolescent mothers drop out of high school.[3]
- When daughters of teen mothers grow up, they are 50 percent more likely to have children before they marry.[4]
- When sons of teen mothers grow up, they are 2.7 times more likely to spend time in prison than the sons of mothers who delay childbearing until their early 20s.[5]

A Familiar Story

Jennifer couldn't believe it when the doctor told her she was pregnant. Sure, she wanted to be a mother someday, but not now. She and Joe had just finished high school. They were so looking forward to college. Her heart pounded and her hands trembled as she started her car. She had to see Joe. He would know what to do.

Tears rolled down her face as she knocked on his front door. Joe immediately knew that something was terribly wrong when he saw Jennifer's face. He stepped outside, reached for Jennifer's hand and said, "What's the matter?"

"We have a problem," she said. "I'm pregnant."

Joe was stunned. His face turned hard. Then he dropped Jennifer's hand and said, "*We* don't have a problem. *You* have a problem." He walked back in the house and shut the door in her face.

Unfortunately, this is an all too familiar story for many young ladies. Girls like Jennifer are devastated by the realization that they are pregnant and left all alone to deal with their situation.

> 2,739 American teenage girls
> get pregnant every day.

Happy Father's Day!

The pain of teenage pregnancy is usually associated with girls. But teenage pregnancies can be very traumatic for the young man as well.

After I finished speaking at a junior high school in Dallas, an eighth grade boy walked up to me and said, "I wish you had spoken to our school last year."

"Why?" I asked.

"Because it's too late for me," he replied.

"Why is it too late?"

"My girlfriend is going to have my baby in three weeks and my life will never be the same again."

My heart broke for this young boy. He looked like the weight of the world was resting on his shoulders. And I guess, in a way, it was. While his friends were thinking about football, baseball and soccer, he was left with the responsibility of fatherhood. I commend him for taking this so seriously, but how sad when today's youth are forced to grow up so fast.

Men: Beware!

Teenage pregnancies are not always accidental. Some girls want to get pregnant. A girl who does not receive enough love and affection at home may be desperate for someone to fill that void.

While a young man may consider her sexual advances no more than a quick fling, she may be making long-term plans. She may believe that if she can get pregnant, he will feel obligated to stay with her. Even if he doesn't stick around, at least she will have a sweet little baby to hold, cuddle, and love. Then, with a blood test, the DNA can prove he is the father. He may then find himself paying child support for the next 18 years. The *CHOICES* he made about a quick little fling have suddenly turned into a nightmare that just won't go away.

Changes in Welfare

Life for a pregnant teenager is tough. But because of recent welfare reform, that life may be much tougher in the very near future. Taxpayers simply will not continue to pay the rising cost of long-term support for those who can't afford to have a baby. The reforms will change long-term support to short-term support, forcing mothers and fathers to become responsible for their families' needs.

Facing the Options

If you were to face an unplanned pregnancy, you would have four options: marriage, single parenting, adoption, or abortion. Of the four *CHOICES*, which one would you choose? Let's consider each.

Marriage

Today, it is rare for young people to choose marriage when facing an unplanned pregnancy. In considering this option, you would have to realize the same thing Chuck and I had to face when we got married: playtime is over! While all our friends were finishing high school, going off to college and having the time of their lives, we had to realize we were no longer two carefree teenagers. We were now a husband and wife, about to become a father and mother with all kinds of responsibilities.

The younger a couple is when they marry, the more likely they are to divorce. Almost one-third of teenage marriages end in divorce within five years, compared to 15 percent of couples who delay marriage until 23 to 29.[6]

I might add that although our parents stood beside Chuck and me and supported us with love, they did not support us financially. No doubt it was difficult and painful for them to watch us struggle. But looking back, it showed great wisdom on their part. Our struggle to pay for Chuck's college, doctor bills and day-to-day expenses forced us to grow up. I believe this is one of the reasons we are still married today. Hard work and responsibility develop character! I believe many parents do their children a great injustice by paying their bills, raising the new baby and allowing their child to continue life as if nothing ever happened.

Single Parenting

In the past few years we have learned a whole new meaning to the term, "Breaking up is hard to do." After going together for two years, Christi and Jake broke up at the end of their senior year in high school. They knew they had to be civilized long enough to sort through all the items they had accumulated during the past two years. They had shared CDs, several computer games, and, oh yes, a baby boy.

When Christi got pregnant her junior year, she was convinced she and Jake would be together forever. When the birth certificate was filled out, Christi gave the baby Jake's last name since they planned to get married within a year. Jake was expecting a nice football scholarship. They would get married, move away, and live happily ever after.

Jake and Christi graduated just as planned. Jake's scholarship was even better than anticipated, but by graduation Jake had a new girlfriend. Jake promised to work each summer and give Christi some money to help with the baby.

Christi is now a single mom to an active three-year-old boy. She still lives at home with her parents but hopes to get her own apartment in the next year or two. She never has made it to college but is considering taking some business classes at night. Although she loves her son, she is sorry she gave him Jake's last name on the birth certificate. It's awkward now having different last names.

Christi dreads it when Jake comes home from college on weekends or holidays. She resents sending her son off to spend time with Jake and his friends and family, but the judge gave Jake visitation rights. Christi hopes Jake will eventually lose interest and get out of their lives.

Yes, breaking up is definitely hard to do these days.

The Reality of Single Parenting

I often speak to an entire class of teenage mothers. This past year I was talking to about 30 teenage girls ranging in ages from 15 to 18. Some were married. Most were single parents. Before the class began, these girls were having fun, laughing and showing off pictures of their cute little babies to all their friends. When the bell rang and the door closed, the laughter stopped and the attitudes changed. As I talked with them and listened to their stories, I asked them what they would say to a group of students who were thinking about having sex. The entire class quickly responded in unison, "Don't do it!" Unfortunately, these young girls learned the hard way that being a teenage mom is not all fun and games.

These girls struggle with a variety of problems. In many cases, the girl's mother keeps the baby while the teenage mom continues her active life of school, work and friends. Grandma's smiling face greets the baby each morning. She's the one who feeds, bathes, and cuddles the child. This setup seems to work well until the baby cries for grandma and not for mommy. The teenage mom's attitude quickly shifts to resentment as she watches her child bonding to her own mother.

This resentment often leads to drastic measures. One 17 year old told me she was desperate to find a man to move in with so she could get out of her parent's house. Unfortunately, men often lose interest in these girls once they learn about "THE BABY." And then there is the other extreme, when girls have lost all trust and respect for men and refuse to get involved in another relationship. The fact that she is a single mother adds a variety of complications to her life not to mention her child's life.

Adoption

Many teenagers have a poor opinion of adoption. They think of it as the ultimate form of rejection.

When speaking to teenagers, I let them know I believe it would be very difficult to carry a baby to full term and then place it for adoption. But I also believe it is an incredible example of sacrificial love when a girl or a young couple says, "We love this baby so much that we want to give it life. But let's be realistic. What kind of life can we give this child?" They then go out and find a family, perhaps a family who cannot have children, and let them raise this baby. Easy? *NO*! But an incredible form of sacrificial love!

Through the years I have worked with hundreds of pregnant teenage girls. One of the most memorable was a 16-year-old girl who told me she often wondered why her birth mother placed her for adoption. She was plagued with the question, "Why didn't she love me enough to keep me?" As we discussed her options regarding her own teenage pregnancy, tears rolled down her face as she said, "Now I understand. My birth mother loved me so *much* that she placed me for adoption."

Through a great deal of pain and many tears, that young girl placed her baby for adoption with a couple who could not have children. The *CHOICE* was not easy! Although she can now finish high school, go on to college, and fulfill other dreams and goals, she will NEVER be able to erase the fact that she is a mother. Somewhere in this world she has a child. But despite the inner pain, she will always know that as a result of her sacrifice she created a family.

A few years ago a young man told me he wanted to find his birth mother just so he could say thank you. He wanted her to know how much he appreciated the sacrifice she had made 18 years earlier, placing him in such a wonderful loving home.

If you are adopted, stop and think about how special you are. Your birth mother did not have to give you life, and your adoptive parents did not have to take you into their home as their own child. Although you may never know all the circumstances that caused your birth mother to place you for adoption, it was no doubt a very difficult and painful situation for her. Adoption is *not* an easy *CHOICE*, but it is an incredible form of sacrificial love!

Abortion

This has been a hot subject for many years. No matter where you stand regarding abortion, we would all agree that no woman looks forward to an abortion. It can be a very painful procedure both physically and emotionally.

At the end of a high school presentation, a school counselor asked if I could speak to a young girl in her office. Upon entering the room I found a 16-year-old girl crying. She told me her parents were divorced and no one in the world loved her. A young man at school recently started coming on to her. The attention made her feel special. When he offered to take her home from school she accepted. When he kissed her, she passionately kissed him back. When he said he wanted to make love to her, she gave herself to him freely. "After all," she said, "that's how they do it in the movies! It's always so beautiful and romantic."

Tears rolled down her face as she continued, "But it wasn't beautiful. It was cheap and dirty, and it hurt a lot. I got pregnant. He left me. I had an abortion and it was also painful. Now all I have are painful memories." She looked so desperate as she said, "I'm worse off now than ever before."

Reflecting Back

I often ask myself what I would have done if abortion had been legal when I was a teenager. What if, back when Chuck and I were scared to death and convinced our lives were about to be destroyed, someone had simply said, "Did you know you can have this problem removed for just a few hundred dollars? And best of all, your parents will never have to know! It can be your secret. Later on if you two want to get married, you can. But don't let this baby be the thing that destroys your life, dreams and goals."

I truly believe with all the fears we had, if someone had told us there was an easy escape, I would have been like so many girls I know today who say, "I hate abortion. I think it's wrong, but I don't have any other *CHOICE*."

If Chuck and I had chosen abortion back then, that little girl I had one month after I graduated from high school would not be alive now. But today, Shannan is a beautiful, 30-year-old woman. She graduated from college in three and a half years with a 4.0 grade point average. Throughout her life she has brought our entire family so much joy and happiness! She has been married to her husband, Brad, for eight years. In the last five years they have blessed us with two precious grandsons, Will and Riley (and one more on the way.) These little boys have brought us so much joy and happiness! It hurts each time I look at my daughter and think, "I could have had her aborted." What a tragedy that would have been!

Abortion can be a painful *CHOICE* and perhaps impossible to be linked with happy memories.

Difficult *CHOICES*

A lady once shared with me that when she was 16 she got pregnant and she reluctantly placed her child for adoption. Two years later she got pregnant again. This time she chose abortion.

A few years later she met a wonderful man and they were married. Soon they were ready to start their family. Shortly after she got pregnant, she had a miscarriage. Then she had another miscarriage and another. The doctor said they were the result of complications from her abortion.

As the lady continued her story, tears ran down her face as she said, "You know if I could go back and change just one thing in my life, it would not be the baby I placed for adoption. It wouldn't even be aborting my second child. If I could change just one thing in my life, I would go back and save myself for my husband on our wedding night. How different my life would be today. The pain and the horrible memories I deal with every day of my life would not be there if only I had waited."

So, which would you choose: marriage, single parenting, adoption, or abortion? Are any of these *CHOICES* easy? Those who choose sexual abstinence until marriage will be free to fulfill their dreams and goals with no fear of a pregnancy before marriage. The *CHOICE* is yours!

At this time complete **Workbook Chapter 5** beginning on the next page.

What Would You Do?

1. If you were involved in a pregnancy in high school, would it be easy to fulfill the dreams and goals you listed in Workbook Chapter 1 (see questions 1 and 2)? Explain.

   _____

   _____

   _____

2. If you were involved in an unplanned pregnancy before marriage, what would be your first reaction?

   _____

   _____

   _____

3. What do you think your parents' first reaction would be?

   _____

   _____

   _____

4. Compare your answer to question #3 to question #8 in Workbook Chapter 2. Which would you prefer?

   _____

   _____

   _____

159

5.   List three people you could turn to for help if you were involved in a pregnancy.

       A._____

       B._____

       C._____

6.   Write down in order of preference which option you would choose if you were involved in a teenage pregnancy. Explain why you would choose that order.

       A._____

       B._____

       C._____

       D._____

       Explanation of order: _____

       _____

       _____

7.   Go to Lori's List in your Workbook Chapter 2. See if you have anything new to add.

Family Discussion

1.   At the end of chapter 4 under the section, "More than Just Me," Marilyn made the following statement: "It's strange. When I chose to become sexually involved, I thought it was just about me. After all, it was a game I decided to play. It was *my* virginity and *my* reputation on the line. Later I began to realize how self-centered I had been." Is having sex really just about the two people involved in the relationship? How could a pregnancy affect the couple's

      A.   parents

      B.   brothers and sisters

      C.   friends

      D.   the baby

2.   In what ways does an unplanned teenage pregnancy create hardships for a teenage girl? How can it impact a boy?

3.   Why do you suppose most teenage boys today choose not to be involved after the girl gets pregnant? Is that right or wrong?

Additional Discussion

⇒ Share with your child the options most teens chose when they faced a pregnancy when you were a teenager. What struggles did they deal with?

⇒ Ask your child the following question: "Now that we have been talking about this, what do you think my reaction would be if you were involved in a pregnancy before marriage?"

References

[1]The Alan Guttmacher Institute, *Sex and the American Teenager*, New York, NY, 1994; 41.

[2]Maynard, Rebecca A., *Kids Having Kids: A Robin Hood Foundation Special Report on the Costs of Adolescent Childbearing*, Robin Hood Foundation: New York, 1996.

[3]Ibid.

[4]Ibid.

[5]Ibid

[6]The Alan Guttmacher Institute, New York, *Sex and America's Teenagers,* 1994; 60.

Note to Parents

You may be surprised by some of the information in the next three chapters dealing with sexually transmitted diseases. Brace yourself, things have changed a great deal since you were a teenager! We are now dealing with a great deal more than syphilis and gonorrhea, and a quick trip to the doctor for a round of penicillin is no longer the easy answer for today's STDs.

One of the most often asked questions by teenagers is, "Why does marriage protect a person from STDs?" The experiment in the Additional Discussion will allow you and your children to have fun as you find the answer to this question. Help your children understand that the secret to being free from STDs is a "Faithfully Committed Lifetime Relationship."

A Tip from the Tool Box:

Tool #2 states, *"CHOICES That Lead to Lifelong Success* require Learning from Those with Experience." Why not apply that tool to parenting? Find a couple who has successfully raised their children and learn from their experience. Talk to them extensively about what they feel they did right and what they wish they had done differently.

Chapter 6

UNDERSTANDING THE
STD EPIDEMIC

Today, those who *CHOOSE* to enter the lifestyle of casual sexual activity walk into an explosive minefield. The mines are not canisters or shells buried underground, but sexually transmitted diseases (STDs).

If your parents grew up in the '60s or '70s, they probably gave little thought to STDs. Syphilis and gonorrhea were the only two common diseases, and both could be cured with antibiotics. Today, you are growing up in the midst of an epidemic of bacterial infections and incurable viruses.

As you search for the secret of *SENSATIONAL SEX* consider the following facts:

Facts:
- There are more than 25 significant STDs.[1]
- Fifteen million Americans are infected with an STD every year.[2]
- Three million teenagers get a new STD every year – 8,219 every day.[3]
- Approximately two-thirds of people who acquire STDs in the U.S. are younger than 25.[4]
- By age 24, at least one in three sexually active people are estimated to have an STD.[5]
- About one out of four sexually active teenagers will get an STD each year.[6]
- The U.S. spends approximately $10 billion each year on major STDs, not including HIV/AIDS. If HIV is included the cost is $17 billion.[7]

The next three chapters will help you understand the current epidemic of sexually transmitted diseases. They will describe in detail several of our nation's leading STDs, including their symptoms, complications, and treatments. You will learn how STDs spread and how they are treated. You will find out which diseases are treatable and which are incurable. You will also gain information as you consider the *CHOICES* that lead to lifelong success.

How STDs Spread

Sexually transmitted diseases are not spread by casual contact. You are not going to get an STD from a cough or a sneeze or by hugging someone. There is no need to worry about getting STDs by eating in restaurants, talking on public telephones, or drinking from a water fountain. It would be rare (but not completely impossible) to become infected by kissing.

Germs from STDs are generally very fragile and die quickly when exposed to air. That's why getting a disease from a toilet seat would also be extremely rare. To survive, the germs must have warmth and moisture.

So how do people get STDs? Usually, they become infected by having sexual intercourse with an infected person. Other risky behaviors, however, can also lead to STDs.

Risky Behavior

Many young people today are involved in passionate relationships, but they stop the physical activity just prior to sexual intercourse. They do this as a means of protection from pregnancy and so they can still call themselves **virgins**. This is commonly called **mutual masturbation**, **outer course**, or **dry sex**.

Couples engaging in this activity might touch under clothing or lie down together without any clothes on. They might bathe or shower together and never consider any of this risky behavior. Are these couples free from worries? NO! Is this risky behavior? YES! Could they be spreading STDs? YES! Just by touching the infected area or sharing bodily fluids a disease can be transmitted in either a **heterosexual** or **homosexual** relationship.

Anal sex and oral sex are also risky behavior. In fact, many STDs are more easily spread by anal intercourse than by vaginal intercourse because of small tears to the rectum.[8] Remember, germs need warmth and moisture to grow. Therefore, both the mouth and rectum are great environments for growing STD germs. The germs from oral sex could result in sores in and around the mouth and throat area.

WARNING: If you are serious about avoiding STDs, you should be careful what you touch and what you kiss.

No Fear of STDs

Not everyone is at risk for STDs. Couples who *CHOOSE* to save sex until they make a lifelong faithful commitment have total sexual freedom! This is called **mutual monogamy**, which means one lifetime partner, or simply put, marriage. Those who are faithful to one lifetime partner are FREE to enjoy sexual intimacy with NO FEAR of STDs.

Some people think they are monogamous because they only have one sexual partner *at a time*. Having five partners in five years is *not* monogamy; it is having multiple sexual partners. It is also very risky behavior and could easily result in STDs.

Warning for Women

Women tend to have more problems with STDs than men. There is a logical explanation for this. The genital area of a woman is warm and moist. Remember, warmth and moisture make the perfect environment for the growth of germs. These germs thrive in the vaginal area and can continue on into the woman's bloodstream.

A teenage girl has a far greater risk of STDs than anyone else. The lining of her cervix, which is the opening to her uterus, is highly susceptible to STDs. Once she reaches her mid-twenties her cervix will undergo a change and will become tougher. Although she can still get STDs, she isn't as vulnerable as a teenage girl.

Warning signs of STDs

Although STDs have a wide variety of symptoms, it is important to know that most people infected with STDs are **asymptomatic**. This is a medical term which simply means they have no signs or symptoms, but they are still contagious. And their condition may be very serious.

> Up to 85 percent of those infected with
> certain STDs are asymptomatic.
>
> No Signs
> No Symptoms
> But Still Contagious[9]

It might be weeks, months, years, or decades before the person knows about the infection.[10] A person can have an STD, be highly contagious, and have no idea anything is wrong.

When symptoms do appear, they are often in the form of sores, a rash, enlarged lymph nodes, pain or a burning sensation while urinating, or severe abdominal pain. Obviously, these symptoms could be attributed to a wide variety of problems besides STDs. A person should never ignore such symptoms but should always consult a doctor for proper treatment.

Help for Those Concerned

If someone you know has been involved in risky behavior, they can choose to change their lifestyle and avoid additional problems. You should encourage them to see a physician because many STDs have treatments and cures. However, the longer a disease goes untreated, the greater the chance of permanent damage.

Go to your workbook and complete **Workbook Chapter 6.**

Test Your Knowledge

1. There are more than _____ significant STDs today.

2. Approximately how many teenagers get an STD every day? _____

3. If you make skin to skin contact with someone's genital area and they have an STD, you can become infected.

    True   False

4. Most people know if they have an STD.   True   False

5. Who has the greatest risk of STDs?_____

6. Asymptomatic means: No _____
    No _____
    But _____

7. Couples who choose to have only one lifetime sexual partner are free to enjoy sexual intimacy with no fear of STDs.

    True   False

8. Explain what "risky behavior" is.

    _____

    _____

    _____

9. If Lori has sex with Brian, is that risky behavior? Explain. (Note: Think about how many sexual partners Brian has had.)

    _____

    _____

169

10. Look back over Lori's List. Add any information Lori should know about STDs before choosing to have sex with Brian.

Family Discussion

1. Check the answers to the Workbook questions in the back of this book.

2. Why is it significant that up to 85 percent of those infected with STDs are asymptomatic?

3. Discuss why teenage girls are at a greater risk for STDs.

4. If a couple is determined that they won't go "all the way" and they take off their clothes and then stop just before sexual intercourse, are they safe? Explain.

5. If a person has three partners in a year, is that risky behavior? If a person has three partners in his or her lifetime, is that risky behavior? Explain.

6. Who are the people with no fear of STDs? Explain.

Additional Discussion

⇒ Try the following experiment. It will help explain how STDs spread. It will also explain the difference between mutual monogamy and multiple sexual partners.

You will need the following items:

6 large drinking glasses
Water
1 tablespoon of clear vinegar

Step 1 – Line the glasses up in a straight row and fill each glass one-third full of water. Each glass represents a person.

Step 2 – Pour the clear vinegar in the first glass. The vinegar represents the infection of a sexually transmitted disease.

Step 3 – Now pour all the liquid from the first glass into the second glass, then return half the liquid back to the first glass.

Step 4 – Repeat the procedure, but this time use glasses two and three.

Step 5 – Now repeat this procedure again using glasses one and four.

QUESTIONS:

     A. Which glasses are now contaminated?

     B. Would you know just by looking at the glasses that they are contaminated?

     C. Do most people with STDs appear to have a problem?

     D. Why aren't glasses five and six contaminated?

Step 6 – Now pour glass five into glass six and return half the water back to glass five again. Repeat that step one more time.

QUESTIONS:

     A. Are glasses five and six contaminated now or do they still contain pure water? Explain.

B. If you poured the water from five and six back and forth 50 times, would they become contaminated or would they still contain pure water? Explain.

C. What has this experiment taught you about multiple sexual partners?

D. What has it taught you about people who save sex for marriage?

When a couple makes the *CHOICE* to save sex for marriage they have total sexual freedom! They can enjoy sex with each other as often as they want and never worry about STDs. Just like the pure water in glasses five and six, you will be sexually pure if you wait until marriage.

QUESTION:

A. What do you hope your future spouse is doing about sex right now:

◊   Saving sex for marriage?

◊   Experimenting with multiple sexual partners?

References

[1] Institute of Medicine, Editors: Thomas R. Eng and William T. Butler, Committee on Prevention and Control of Sexually Transmitted Diseases, *The Hidden Epidemic: Confronting Sexually Transmitted Diseases*, National Academy Press, Washington, D.C., 1997; 1.

[2] Kaiser Family Foundation and American Social Health Association, *STDs in America: How Many Cases and At What Cost?* Menlo Park, CA; 1998;4.

[3] Ibid.

[4] Ibid.

[5] Ibid.

[6] Kaiser Family Foundation and American Social Health Association, *STDs in America: How Many Cases and At What Cost?* Menlo Park, CA; 1998; 10.

[7] Institute of Medicine, *The Hidden Epidemic: Confronting Sexually Transmitted Diseases*, 1997; 1.

[8] Ibid., 72.

[9] Ibid., 70.

[10] Ibid.

Note to Parents

When people think of STDs today, they usually think about AIDS. As you are about to learn, there are many more problems than AIDS. One major problem with today's STDs is that they can leave a person sterile. I heard a doctor recently say that the teenagers of today are going to be known as the sterile society because of the complications from many of today's sexually transmitted diseases. As a parent, you cannot make *CHOICES* for your children. You are, however, responsible for giving them good information. The medical information they will receive in these chapters can have a great impact on their future, dreams and goals.

As a word of warning, the information can be frightening. You may want to remind your children that this is not a fear message. It is a freedom message. Those who choose sexual abstinence are *FREE* from all the problems described in these chapters. It is only those going from partner to partner who have to worry about such problems.

After speaking on a college campus I had some students approach me in anger. When I asked them why they were angry, they responded, "Because no one ever told us all this stuff about the diseases before today. We can handle the truth, if people will just tell us the truth."

Your children deserve to know the truth about today's STD epidemic.

A Tip from the Tool Box:

> If you are out of town or out late because of a meeting, take a break and call your child. Ask about his or her day and tell them that you miss them. Young people who feel connected with their parents are more likely to postpone sex.

Chapter 7

COMMON CURABLE STDs

Many STDs are bacterial infections. These STDs can generally be cured with proper medication. Time, however, is of the essence. Bacterial infections can be extremely destructive if not treated before they have caused damage. This chapter will provide detailed information, statistics, and true stories of individuals who have been infected with some of the leading bacterial STDs.

Chlamydia

According to the Centers for Disease Control and Prevention (CDC), chlamydia is the most common bacterial STD in the U.S. Over three million Americans develop a new chlamydia infection each year. Most of these infections are among teenagers and young adults. In fact some studies indicate that up to 30 to 40 percent of sexually active teenage girls are infected with chlamydia.[1] However, 85 percent of the females and 40 percent of the males who have this infection are asymptomatic: no signs, no symptoms, but still contagious.[2] Chlamydia may remain silent in the reproductive system for days, months, or years, yet the damage can be devastating.

If women develop symptoms, they usually include a discharge, painful burning with urination, and urgency or frequency of urination. They may also experience pain in the lower abdomen and fever. Symptoms for men include a discharge of pus from the penis and painful burning with urination.

The greatest danger of chlamydia is that it can cause an infection in the female's uterus, fallopian tubes, and ovaries. This is called **pelvic inflammatory disease (PID)**. Chlamydia PID can destroy a woman's reproductive system without her being aware of

177

any problems. The damage may make it extremely difficult or impossible for her to get pregnant. This is why chlamydia is now being labeled the silent sterilizer.

A man with chlamydia may also become **infertile**; however, in most cases the damage will not be permanent and can be reversed with medication.

Diagnosis and Treatment

It is critical for both sexual partners to be treated for chlamydia to ensure it is not passed back and forth. A doctor can diagnose chlamydia by testing secretions from the woman's cervix or the man's penis. If chlamydia is detected, a doctor can prescribe medication to cure the infection, but the damage from the infection may be permanent. Therefore, early detection is critical.

Impact to Children

Chlamydia can cause miscarriages, premature births, and tubal pregnancies. More than 100,000 babies are born with chlamydia each year. However, the baby will not have chlamydia or fertility problems like the mother but is at risk of developing serious eye infections or middle ear infections. The baby is also at risk of developing pneumonia.[3]

A True Story

Stacy was a 24-year-old college student who shared her personal story after I spoke on her college campus. She said she and her husband had recently decided they were ready to start their family. She went to the doctor for a check-up to make sure everything was okay. After the examination and several tests the doctor said, "I'm sorry to tell you, but there really isn't any hope of your having a child." He went on to explain, "You have had chlamydia PID so severely in the past that it has destroyed your reproductive system. Perhaps you and your husband will want to begin considering adoption."

She looked at me with tears rolling down her face and said, "The sad thing is, I NEVER knew I had a sexually transmitted disease. I never knew anything was wrong until the doctor told me I couldn't conceive and have children with my husband."

She explained she had only had three sexual partners in her life: one in high school, one in her freshman year in college, and then her husband. She never thought of three partners as a risky lifestyle. After all, some of her friends had three or more partners a year, and they didn't have any problems. Or did they? Perhaps, like Stacy, they are just beginning to receive the damage reports from having multiple sexual partners.

Gonorrhea

Ask a group of people to name as many STDs as possible. No doubt, gonorrhea would be near the top of their list. Most people know of this disease, but few know of the problems it creates.

Gonorrhea is a pus-producing bacterium which is transmitted almost exclusively through sexual intercourse. Teenage girls ages 15 to 19 have the highest rates of gonorrhea in the U.S.[4] A man or woman may be infected with gonorrhea and be asymptomatic for days or months and yet still be highly contagious. Eventually, this infection usually begins to cause pain and obvious symptoms.

When symptoms do develop, they include a pus-like discharge for both men and women. The infection can also cause frequent urination, or it can make urination impossible. In this case, a woman may require catheterization (a tube inserted into her urinary tract to enable urination). Men may require a similar procedure in the urethra to allow urination and ejaculation.

Gonorrhea can also move into the bloodstream of both men and women and then into the joints, resulting in septic arthritis. This can be cured with intensive antibiotic therapy, but it may leave permanent scarring in the joints.[5]

The greatest danger of gonorrhea for women is PID, which can result in **sterility** or **tubal pregnancies**. Gonorrhea PID may produce such severe chronic pelvic pain that women will welcome a **hysterectomy**, the surgical removal of the uterus.

Diagnosis and Treatment

When a person is tested for STDs, doctors usually check for both chlamydia and gonorrhea. If a person has one of these diseases they often have the other one as well. The doctor can culture secretions from the man's penis or a woman's vaginal area to check for gonorrhea. If the test comes back positive, the doctor will usually begin treatment by using antibiotics.

This sounds easy enough, but now there are antibiotic-resistant strains of gonorrhea.[6] This does not mean these new strains cannot be cured. It just means the medication may cost significantly more and valuable time may be lost trying to find the right cure. The longer a person has gonorrhea the greater the chance of permanent damage.

It is important that both partners are treated and cured so they will not continue to pass the infection back and forth to each other.

Impact to Children

Gonorrhea does not cause PID and infertility problems for a newborn, but it may cause serious eye infections for the baby which may result in blindness. That is why newborns are routinely treated with eye drops to prevent infection.

A True Story

A nurse shared the story of a 17-year-old football player who entered the emergency room around midnight. His knee was extremely swollen and he was in severe pain. After the fluid was drained off the swollen joint, the tests revealed an arthritic infection from gonorrhea. The young man was admitted to the hospital for a few days for an intravenous antibiotic treatment. Who would ever think a swollen knee could be the result of an STD?

Pelvic Inflammatory Disease – PID

Pelvic inflammatory disease, commonly called PID, is not a sexually transmitted disease. It is, however, one of the most common complications of STDs. These problems only affect females and are the result of an infection in the uterus, fallopian tubes, or ovaries. A girl or woman usually gets PID from chlamydia or gonorrhea.[7]

More than one million American women have complications from PID every year.[8] This infection can leave a woman infertile, making it difficult or impossible for her to ever become pregnant. There are many reasons why a couple might not be able to have children, but about 30 percent of such cases result from sexually transmitted diseases which cause PID.[9]

PID may result in fever and severe abdominal pain, pain while exercising, or pain during sexual intercourse. PID may also be asymptomatic. The infection can be equally damaging with or without pain. The unsuspecting woman may never know she has a problem until she is ready to begin her family and nothing happens.

Because of PID, many teenage girls and women require major surgery to remove an ovary or fallopian tube. In the more severe cases, a hysterectomy is required to remove the uterus. About 30,000 American women undergo hysterectomies each year because of PID.[10]

A potentially fatal complication of PID is tubal (or ectopic) pregnancies. In a tubal pregnancy, the fertilized egg becomes lodged in the scarred fallopian tube. This can result in severe hemorrhaging. It is estimated that tubal pregnancies have increased 500 percent in the past twenty years.[11]

Syphilis

Syphilis is another common STD that everyone seems to recognize. This disease has plagued nations for centuries, tormenting young and old, rich and poor.

While everyone seems to have heard of syphilis, few people know the actual symptoms. It can be transmitted both through sexual intercourse and skin-to-skin contact with the infected area. While easily treated, it can be fatal if left untreated.

Stages of Syphilis

Syphilis infections progress through three separate stages.

First stage: Primary syphilis occurs within a few days or several weeks of sexual contact with an infected person. The first symptom is a painless sore called a chancre (pronounced "shanker"). It appears where the infection invaded the body: in the genital area, in the mouth, or on the lips. This painless sore disappears after two to eight weeks even if left untreated.

Second stage: Secondary syphilis appears six weeks to six months later. Symptoms may include headaches, fever, fatigue, enlarged lymph nodes, and skin rashes. During this stage a person is most contagious. The symptoms will clear up after a few weeks or months even without treatment.

Final stage: The last stage of syphilis can eventually be life-threatening, and the damage can become irreversible. This stage may not occur for several months or up to twenty years. Almost any part of the body can be attacked, producing severe damage to the brain, heart, blood vessels, nervous system, bones, or skin.[12]

Diagnosis and Treatment

Syphilis can be difficult to identify. Doctors diagnose it through a blood test, but it may take up to six months after a person is infected for a blood test to appear positive. Once detected, however, this STD can generally be completely cured by adequate doses of antibiotics.

A painless sore anywhere in the genital or mouth area should not go unchecked. This could be syphilis! One of the greatest concerns is that syphilis greatly increases the susceptibility to being infected with HIV.[13]

Impact to Children

The greatest tragedy of syphilis is what it can do to unborn children. A mother can actually give syphilis to the baby while it is still inside her womb. Many of these pregnancies will result in spontaneous miscarriages or stillbirths. Of those who survive the birth process, many are infected and die soon after birth. Babies who survive often have serious abnormalities.[14]

A True Story

At the conclusion of a program in a high school, a 17-year-old boy told me he had a severe rash. "Could this be associated with an STD?" he asked.

I told him the only way to know for sure was to go to a doctor. After all, a rash could result from many different problems. I did tell him, however, that the second stage of syphilis is often associated with a rash. For that reason, it would be worth going to the doctor to have it checked.

Later that day, the school counselor informed me that several students in the school had syphilis. I hope that young man took my advice and went to the doctor. If the rash resulted from syphilis, it could be easily treated at this stage. If he lets it go, it will soon disappear. He will never know anything is wrong until he is diagnosed with a severe heart condition or perhaps life-threatening complications of the brain or nervous system.

Crabs

Crabs is not a bacterial infection. It is actually a slang term for pubic lice. I have included it here because I've had so many teenagers ask me what it is. Here's the answer. Pubic lice are tiny creatures that will not kill you but can be very annoying! They do little harm other than cause intense itching and irritation of the skin in the pubic (genital) area of men and women.

Pubic lice are usually transmitted by having sexual intercourse or sexual contact with an infected person. They can also be transmitted through contact with the clothing or bed sheets of an infected person.[15]

Diagnosis and Treatment

Pubic lice are visible to the naked eye. A doctor can prescribe a special shampoo to wash the hair around the pubic area to kill the lice. It is important for an infected person to wash all of their bed linens, towels and clothes in hot water.

183

Perhaps you are now beginning to see how the *CHOICES* you make about sex can lead to lifelong success or a lifetime of regrets.

After reviewing the Quick Reference Chart on the next page, go to your workbook and complete **Workbook Chapter 7.**

QUICK REFERENCE CHART FOR CURABLE STDs

STD	Concern	Symptoms
Chlamydia – Most common bacterial STD. 3 million Americans infected yearly.	Can scar the female reproductive system, leaving her infertile. May cause a man to be infertile but he can usually be cured with medication.	85% of women are asymptomatic. Men often experience a discharge of pus and painful burning while urinating.
Gonorrhea – Pus producing bacteria. 650,000 people infected in the U.S. each year.	Can scar the female reproductive system leaving her infertile. May cause a man to be infertile but usually treatable with medication. Can also cause septic arthritis for men and women.	Often asymptomatic at first but most men and women develop a discharge of pus, severe pain, and burning while urinating.
PID – Not an STD but the most common complication of STDs. One million U.S. women develop PID yearly.	Can scar the female reproductive system leaving her infertile. Also increases her chances for a tubal pregnancy, which is always fatal for the baby and can be life-threatening for the girl.	Affects only women. Asymptomatic or severe abdominal pain. Can also cause pain during sexual intercourse.
Syphilis – 3 stages over several years. 70,000 Americans infected yearly.	Can cause permanent damage and death if left untreated through the final stage.	First state – painless sore. Second stage – rash, fever, fatigue, etc. Final stage – permanent damage to heart, brain, etc.
Crabs – Slang for pubic lice.	Causes an annoying itch and skin irritation.	Intense itching in the pubic area resulting in small sores that ooze pus.

Test Your Knowledge

1. Match the STD with the correct symptom.

   A. PID   B. Chlamydia   C. Gonorrhea   D. Syphilis   E. Crabs

   _____ 1. Most common bacterial STD in the U.S.; known as the silent sterilizer.
   _____ 2. Starts with a painless sore and can lead to death if untreated.
   _____ 3. Causes an annoying itch.
   _____ 4. A pus-producing STD.
   _____ 5. Can destroy a woman's uterus, fallopian tubes and ovaries.

2. Which disease or condition discussed in this chapter would concern you most? Why?

   _____

   _____

   _____

   _____

3. Look back over Lori's List. Write down anything you feel you should warn her about.

Family Discussion

1. Check the answers in the back of this book.

2. Which of the diseases discussed in the chapter did you already know about?

3.   Discuss the diseases that concern you the most and explain why.

4.   Why is PID so serious?

5.   From the knowledge you gained from this chapter, explain how *CHOICES* about sex can lead to lifelong regrets.

6.   Review Lori's List and see what new additions have been made.

Additional Discussion

⇒ How do you suppose it would feel to know you or your spouse were sterile because of an STD? How could this cause additional stress in your marriage?

⇒ What problems might a baby have if born to a mother with an STD?

References

[1]Kaiser Family Foundation, American Social Health Association, *Sexually Transmitted Diseases in American: How Many Cases and at What Cost?* Menlo Park, CA., December 1998.

[2]Institute of Medicine, *The Hidden Epidemic: Confronting Sexually Transmitted Diseases*, 1997; 34.

[3]The Alan Guttmacher Institute, *The Facts in Brief*, New York, NY, 1993.

[4]Centers for Disease Control and Prevention. Sexually Transmitted Disease Surveillance 1995. *Morbidity and Mortality Weekly Report*, September 1996.

[5]McIlhaney, Joe S., Jr., M.D., *Sex: What You Don't Know Can Kill You*, Baker Books, 1997; 31.

[6]Handsfield, H.H. and Whittington, W.L., "Antibiotic Resistant Neisseria Gonorrhea: The Calm Before the Storm?" *Annals of Internal Medicine*, September 1996; 125(6), 507-509.

[7]Centers for Disease Control and Prevention. Sexually Transmitted Disease Surveillance 1995. *Morbidity and Mortality Weekly Report*, September 1996.

[8]Rolfs R.T, et al., "Pelvic Inflammatory Disease: Trends in Hospitalizations and Office Visits, 1979 through 1988," *American Journal Obstetrics and Gynecology* 1992; 166:983-90.

[9]Centers for Disease Control and Prevention. Sexually Transmitted Disease Surveillance 1995. Office of Women's Health, Atlanta, GA, 1997.

[10]The Alan Guttmacher Institute, *The Facts in Brief*, New York, NY, 1993.

[11]Centers for Disease Control and Prevention Sexually Transmitted Disease Surveillance 1995. Office of Women's Health, Atlanta, GA, 1997.

[12]McIlhaney, Joe S., Jr., M.D., *Sex: What You Don't Know Can Kill You*, Baker Books, 1997; 49-53.

[13]Centers for Disease Control and Prevention. Sexually Transmitted Disease Surveillance 1995. *Morbidity and Mortality Weekly Report*, September, 1996.

[14]Institute of Medicine, *The Hidden Epidemic: Confronting Sexually Transmitted Diseases*, 1997; 47.

[15]McIlhaney, Joe S., Jr., M.D., *Safe Sex: A Doctor Explains the Realities of AIDS and Other STDs*, Baker House, 1994; 168.

Note to Parents

It is important to help your children understand the complications of asymptomatic diseases. Just because a person looks and feels healthy does not mean they do not have a sexually transmitted disease. People with HIV are usually asymptomatic for several years. They have no signs, no symptoms, but are contagious. The same can be true with any of the viral STDs discussed in this chapter.

Your children will learn in this chapter that condoms will not always prevent STDs. Even if a condom is used consistently and correctly, a person can still get herpes and HPV since these viruses spread throughout the genital area. More information will be given regarding condoms and other contraceptives later in the book.

This chapter concludes by encouraging the young people to tell their parents or the adult who gave them this book if they have any personal concerns about possible STDs. There is a good chance your child has *not* been involved in any type of risky behavior and you will get no response or reaction. However, you do need to be prepared for the possibility that your child may express the need to see a doctor. If this happens, the most important thing you can do is to stay calm. This may not be easy, but realize that it is taking a great deal of courage for your child to share this information. Unconditional love is needed from you at this time, not anger and ridicule.

If your child doesn't share any concerns verbally, watch for nonverbal signs during the family discussion. If your child suddenly seems withdrawn or bothered, try to find out what is concerning him or her.

If you find your child has been involved in risky behavior, contact your family doctor regarding how you should proceed. Then go to the doctor with your child. Let your child know you will always be there for him/her and nothing will stop you from loving him/her.

Tip from the Tool Box:

Wait up for your children when they go out at night. Greet them with a smile and let them tell you all about the evening's events. Your children may think long and hard about getting involved in drugs, alcohol, or sex if they know your smiling face will be greeting them at the door!

Chapter 8

COMMON INCURABLE STDs

Not all sexually transmitted diseases can be cured. Any time you see the word **viral** or **virus** you need to think "no cure." The common cold is a virus and there has never been a cure for it. Although you can take medicine to help some of the symptoms, you can't take a pill to make the cold go away.

Viral STDs are the same way. There is, however, a major difference between the cold virus and STD viruses. When the cold virus runs its course, it goes away. A cold returns only if you catch another cold virus. However, if a person is infected with a viral STD such as herpes, hepatitis B, HPV, or HIV, they can be infected and contagious for life, with or without symptoms.

The following are some of the more common viral STDs.

Herpes

Herpes is a very common virus which produces painful blisters and sores in and around the genital area. One out of five Americans from 12 years of age and up are infected with genital herpes. That is approximately 45 million Americans![1] According to the Herpes Resource Center, victims are usually well-educated and middle to upper class. Although herpes is not a life-threatening disease, it can be annoying, painful, and extremely embarrassing.

About 90 percent of those infected with herpes do not realize they have the disease, yet they can be highly contagious even if the sores are not present.[2] For those who do experience painful sores, outbreaks may occur several times a month or year. They may disappear for years and then suddenly reappear. That is why herpes is known as "the gift that keeps on giving."

Tight clothing (such as jeans) and stress often bring on new sores. Therefore, such activities as cheerleading tryouts, finishing a term paper, preparing for finals, a job interview, or preparation for a wedding might trigger a new outbreak. These are not the times a person would want to deal with painful sores.

It is important to understand that condoms (see glossary for definition) will not always prevent the spread of herpes. Transmission of this virus can occur from skin to skin. The sores can spread throughout the genital area and other parts of the body which are not covered by a condom.[3]

Diagnosis and Treatment

Doctors can usually identify a herpes sore by a simple examination. To confirm the diagnosis, the physician can swab the infected area and grow a culture.

A doctor can prescribe medication in ointment or pill form to help relieve the pain. Although this is not a cure, it often helps control the outbreaks. This medication can be a welcomed relief, however, it is expensive.

Occasionally, men and women with herpes have to be hospitalized. Recently a doctor told me of a 17-year-old girl who had such severe blisters she couldn't urinate. She was admitted into the hospital and catheterized (so she could urinate) and was given morphine for the excruciating pain of the sores.

Impact to Children

Herpes increases the risk of miscarriages and premature deliveries. A baby born to a herpes-infected mother can die or have severe brain damage. Delivering the baby by cesarean section prevents the child from passing through the birth canal and coming into contact with the herpes virus.

A True Story

Mindy was seventeen when she gave her virginity to Kyle, the love of her life. One month later she developed painful blisters around her genital area. She was devastated when her doctor told her she had herpes. By passing this infection on, Kyle enlisted Mindy in the ranks of 45 million other Americans who have herpes.

Although Kyle and Mindy have the same disease, their symptoms have been very different. Mindy experiences painful blisters almost every month. With time the sores may eventually disappear, or Mindy may have them off and on the rest of her life.

Kyle, on the other hand, is asymptomatic. He had no idea he had a sexually transmitted disease until he infected Mindy. He had sex with two other girls before he met Mindy. Obviously, one of those girls had herpes. Kyle may never have an outbreak of the sores, or it might be months or years before they suddenly appear.

Although Kyle and Mindy are not going to die from herpes, they must deal with the emotional pain and embarrassment that they have an incurable sexually transmitted disease.

Unfortunately, Kyle did not end up being the love of Mindy's life. Three months after she contracted herpes, they broke up. Now, Kyle and Mindy have to face the probability of passing this incurable disease on to future sexual partners, including their spouses. Even if they choose abstinence until marriage, I do not envy them having to tell a potential marriage partner that they have herpes, an incurable sexually transmitted disease. Nor do I envy their future spouses, who may be unable to avoid contracting the disease. The effects of Kyle's and Mindy's *CHOICES* certainly are not limited to themselves.

Hepatitis B

This virus was discovered as a sexually transmitted disease only 20 years ago, yet today it is one of the most common STDs in the world. About two-thirds of the total current hepatitis B cases are spread by sexual contact. There are 77,000 new sexually transmitted cases of hepatitis B each year.[4]

Hepatitis B is the most common cause of liver cancer in the U.S. It also causes cirrhosis of the liver. Each year approximately

5,000 Americans die as a result of liver complications from Hepatitis B.[5]

This highly contagious virus is not transmitted through food, water, or casual contact, but only through infected bodily fluids. Although it can be sexually transmitted, anyone around contaminated blood or other bodily fluids is at risk. This would include health care workers, drug addicts, and those living with infected individuals. These people can protect themselves with a hepatitis B vaccine.

A person may have hepatitis B with absolutely no symptoms yet be highly contagious for the rest of his or her life. Those who have symptoms may experience yellowing of the skin and eyes, lack of energy, nausea, vomiting, or dark urine. Although the symptoms usually clear up in a few weeks, the person can remain contagious.

Diagnosis and Treatment

Hepatitis B is diagnosed by a blood test. Although there is no cure for this virus, a vaccine can prevent the infection.

Impact to Children

All pregnant women are encouraged to have a blood test for hepatitis B. If the mother has the virus, the baby can receive a vaccine at birth. Otherwise the baby could become infected, be contagious for life and develop liver cancer.

Human Papilloma Virus (HPV)

HPV is the most common STD in the United States and is becoming a major epidemic among the teenage population. It is estimated that 20 million Americans are already infected with HPV, with 5.5 million new infections occurring each year.[6]

Dr. Hal Wallis, an obstetrician and gynecologist and president of the Texas Physicians Resource Council, recently told me that during his 20 years of practice he has never had a patient who was HIV positive. But a day doesn't go by that he doesn't deal with HPV. He said most of his patients who are infected with HPV are young women 15 to 25 years of age. Dr. Wallis said that he is very concerned about the impact of HPV on today's young people, because like HIV, HPV can be deadly.

This increasing incidence of HPV has been seen in college campuses across the country. A recent study from Rutgers University reported that over a three-year period 60 percent of the females at that university were infected with HPV.[7]

HPV can cause warts inside and around the genital area including the buttocks and crease of the legs. The warts, which resemble a cauliflower, cause little pain but are highly contagious. They are usually small but can grow to be large and uncomfortable.[8]

Treatment of Genital Warts

Doctors usually treat genital warts by burning, freezing, or cutting them off. Often multiple treatments are required which can become very expensive and frustrating. A man told me he had suffered from genital warts for several years. Every few months he went to his doctor to have the warts removed, but they kept coming back. A urologist recently told me the largest genital wart he has treated was on a 23-year-old man. There were actually two warts and both were about the size of a grapefruit. The doctor told me it took three major operations to remove these warts.

Another doctor told me he performed a two-hour laser surgery on an 18-year-old girl to remove over 100 small warts from her genital and buttocks area. He said when he finished, her bottom looked like a worn-out pin cushion. Hopefully, her warts won't come back. But even if the warts don't return, she still has HPV and is contagious.

Additional Problems

Genital warts are not the major problem associated with HPV. The greater concern is that this STD can cause cancer. Cancer from HPV for men is rare. If it occurs, it is cancer of the penis or anus. Cancer for women, unfortunately, is common. This includes cancer of the cervix, vagina and vulva. Cervical cancer kills about 4,900 women in our country every year.[9] A recent study found that HPV causes "virtually all cervical cancers."[10]

As with most other sexually transmitted diseases, an individual can have HPV and have no symptoms. Some people may have the virus for months, years or decades before they are aware of it. Yet every person they have intimate contact with can contract this disease. This contact need not be limited to sexual intercourse; it can be skin to skin contact with the infected area.

Unfortunately, condoms provide little to no protection from HPV.[11] This virus can spread throughout the genital area including the crease of the legs and the buttocks as well as a man's scrotum. A condom does not cover these areas!

Diagnosing and Treating Cancer

A **Pap smear** is a simple test using secretions from the female cervix and vagina to detect early signs of cancer. If the Pap smear indicates precancerous cells, the doctor will either freeze the infected area or treat it with a laser or perform minor surgery. These procedures usually take place in the doctor's office and can be continued for months or years until the Pap smear is normal.

If the Pap smear indicates cancer, aggressive treatment must begin immediately. This requires radical surgery and/or radiation therapy.

All sexually active females must understand the danger of HPV and the importance of Pap smears. As Dr. Laurette Dekat has said, "Once you've passed that magic line [of having sex], you've bought yourself an annual Pap smear for life."[12]

Remember, HPV is a virus. Therefore, there is no cure. Warts can be removed. Precancerous and cancerous cells can possibly be destroyed, but a doctor can do nothing to make this disease go away.

Impact to Children

The treatments for HPV can damage or weaken a woman's cervix, causing infertility and premature births. During pregnancy, the warts have a tendency to multiply rapidly. It is possible for the baby to become infected with HPV while passing through the birth canal. In extreme cases the infant might develop warts on the vocal cords, requiring surgery to remove the warts.

A True Story

A doctor in the Dallas area told me of a 13-year-old girl who came to him because of cancer resulting from HPV. The doctor had to perform two major operations on this young girl, removing a portion of her genital area. Yet, this 13-year-old girl is still a virgin. So how did she get this sexually transmitted disease?

It seems that she had a 15-year-old boyfriend. He had only had sex with one girl before he met the 13 year old. He did not know he had the human papilloma virus. He was asymptomatic – no signs, no symptoms – but he was highly contagious.

One Friday night his parents were gone. He decided to take advantage of the opportunity by asking the 13-year-old girl to come over to his house. They went into his bedroom, laid down on his bed, and began to kiss and hug. As the evening progressed they removed their clothes, but they never had sexual intercourse. However, just the skin-to-skin contact was enough to pass the virus to the young girl – a virus he didn't even know he had.

This young girl had no idea the *CHOICES* she made that evening would result in lifelong consequences. She has now had two operations. She must visit the doctor regularly to keep close check on possible future complications. She will also have to live with the fact that she can infect any future sexual partner with this STD.

Let's not forget the young man who infected her. Is he still contagious? Yes. Even though he may never have any signs or symptoms, he can infect every person that comes into sexual contact with him, including his future wife. How horrible for a man to realize the *CHOICES* he made about having a little fun on a Friday night resulted in cancer and perhaps the death of his past girlfriends and his wife.

Don't forget, this is the fastest spreading STD in America.

AIDS (Acquired Immune Deficiency Syndrome)

AIDS, which is caused by HIV (human immunodefiency virus) was discovered in 1981. At that time there were only a small number of known cases in the United States. Today, there are about 900,000 living Americans who are infected with HIV.[13] Of those infected, 560,000 were infected through sexual transmission.[14] That means approximately one out of every 300 Americans over the age of 13 now has HIV.[15]

By 1998, over 375,000 Americans had died of AIDS.[16] As a comparison, about 56,000 Americans died during the Vietnam War. In 1994, AIDS became the leading cause of death of American men and women between the ages of 25 and 44.

HIV is transmitted through the exchange of bodily fluids. This usually happens through sexual activity, sharing contaminated needles, or through blood transfusions. For years, AIDS was considered a problem almost exclusively for homosexuals and drug users. Today, that profile is changing. Heterosexual relationships (girl-guy relationships) now represent the fastest growing proportion of AIDS cases in the U.S.[17]

There is a major link between HIV and the other STDs. The sores and inflammation produced by herpes, syphilis, HPV, hepatitis B, gonorrhea, and chlamydia greatly increase the chance of HIV infection.

Within four to eight weeks after contracting HIV, a person might have the symptoms of mononucleosis. These last only a short time before the symptoms disappear. Although the person can look and feel healthy for a number of years, they will probably be infected and contagious for life.

As HIV progresses, people often begin to experience enlarged lymph nodes, fever, weight loss, diarrhea, candida mouth infections, and shingles. When these symptoms occur, the person is said to have AIDS. As the immune system weakens, infections such as pneumonia, non-Hodgkin's lymphoma, and Kaposi's Sarcoma (the most common AIDS-related tumor) often begin to invade the body. Within a year of these symptoms, 50 percent of infected persons will die. About 90 percent will die within three years. This is why AIDS has been labeled by many experts as an almost perfect killing machine.[18]

Impact to Children

About 6,000 babies are born to HIV-infected women every year. The good news is 75 percent of babies born to HIV-positive mothers will not become HIV positive. If the mother is treated with AZT during her pregnancy, there is only an 8 percent chance that the baby will be HIV positive. Unfortunately, those children who do contract HIV from their mothers usually do not live past the age of four.[19]

Diagnosis and Treatment

AIDS is diagnosed through a blood test. Although a person is contagious, tests will not appear positive for at least three to six months after the initial infection.

Scientists around the world are working diligently to find a cure or vaccine for AIDS. This is going to be difficult, perhaps impossible, because there are already over 150 strains of this disease. Remember, there has NEVER been a cure for any known virus, not even the common cold.

The past few years have seen some major breakthroughs in suppressing the viral activity of AIDS and controlling many of its complications. Doctors can count the number of viruses in the bloodstream and monitor the patient's responses to treatment. While these drugs have significantly improved the health of many AIDS patients, they are very expensive. This medication costs about $20,000 a year. Since the drugs are toxic, they often make the patient extremely ill. Many patients cannot tolerate the side effects and have to stop taking them. While these treatments can improve and prolong the life of AIDS patients, they are NOT a cure.

A True Story

The following true story was written by Christina Stuart. It appeared in the S.E. Polk Community District School newspaper, *The Unifier*, in Iowa on April 19, 1996.

To high school kids everywhere:
. . . On December 17, 1995, one of my best friends, Meggan, died at the age of 17 of Kaposi's Sarcoma, which is a cancer found in AIDS patients. Meggan had only had sex twice in her life and one of these killed her. Meggan was not a typical AIDS patient. It only took her two years to become infected, develop full-blown AIDS, and

die. She was a caring person and a best friend to many. She did not deserve to die.

I talked to the guy who gave her the disease. He didn't know that he was infected at the time he gave it to Meggan, and he told me repeatedly how sorry he was for "killing" her. He feels so bad that he is still healthy and alive – and she is gone. It doesn't happen very often that the person who passes on this disease lives to feel the pain and remorse of seeing the results of their carelessness. He lives each day knowing that very soon he will be joining her.

Now I come to the real shocker of my story. They were using a condom at the time she got infected. Do you see what I'm getting at? No matter how "safe" you're being, if you're having sex you are putting yourself in danger. Because of AIDS, sex can KILL!!!!

Most high school students won't have a story like mine until much later in their lives. AIDS takes years, in typical cases, to surface and more time after that to kill. How long will it be before your Meggan dies? How many lives have to be wasted before we realize that the key to stopping this is within each one of us? I wouldn't wish my pain, Meggan's pain, or her infector's pain on anyone. Stop having sex before you and the people you love have to experience this pain. Don't become another statistic. Together we can stop the cycle here before anyone else has to die, physically or emotionally. Think about it. It can happen to you.

With so much love,
Your big sister

And Now – The Rest of the Story

I recently contacted Christina, the young lady who wrote that letter, and asked for an update on Meggan's boyfriend. She informed me that Jacob passed away on May 5, 1998 from pneumonia caused by complications of the AIDS virus. She said Jacob lived for two and a half years knowing that not only was he going to die, but that he was responsible for Meggan's death.

Christina said she and Jacob went through some rough times, but in the end they became friends. Now Christina has lost two friends to AIDS, two young people who made the *CHOICE* to trust their lives to a condom.

Conclusion

Only those who have exchanged bodily fluids or had skin to skin contact with the infected area of a person with an STD have to be concerned about getting one of these diseases. If you have never had intimate contact with another person you have NO FEAR of STDs. If you have been involved in any type of risky behavior, please talk to your parents or the person who gave you this book. They obviously care about you and want to help.

Testing for STDs

Most doctors recommend a person be tested for chlamydia and gonorrhea within one month after each new sexual partner. Tests for hepatitis B, syphilis, and HIV should also be taken, but it is best to wait six months after the initial sexual encounter. Tests taken earlier than six months may come back negative when they are actually positive.

Doctors do not normally test for herpes or HPV, because there is nothing the doctor can do even if the person has the virus. Doctors do, however, encourage all women and all sexually active girls to have yearly Pap smears to detect any abnormal cells that can lead to cancer as a result of HPV. In other words, girls should start having annual pelvic exams as soon as they start having sexual contact. After all, a girl's fertility and life are at risk.

CHOICES

The *CHOICES* you make about sex can have a profound impact on your future. Those *CHOICES* are not just about you. They are also about your future spouse and children. Your *CHOICES* can lead to lifelong success or a lifetime of regret.

After reviewing the Quick Reference Chart on the next page, complete **Workbook Chapter 8**.

QUICK REFERENCE CHART FOR INCURABLE STDs

STD	Concern	Symptoms
Herpes – 45 million Americans estimated to have herpes with 1 million new infections each year.	No cure. Herpes-infected babies can die or have serious problems. Condoms do not always prevent this STD.	Many are asymptomatic, but others have painful blisters in the genital area off and on throughout their life.
Hepatitis B – 750,000 Americans are infected from sexual transmission with 77,000 new cases each year.	No cure. There is, however, a vaccine for prevention. The most common cause of liver cancer. Kills 5,000 Americans a year.	Many are asymptomatic, but there may be a yellowing of the eyes and skin, nausea, vomiting, and dark urine.
HPV – Most common STD. 20 million Americans are infected with 5.5 million new infections each year.	No cure. Over 4,900 American women die each year from HPV associated cancer. Warts are highly contagious. Condoms give little or no protection from this STD	Many are asymptomatic, but some will develop genital warts.
AIDS – Caused by HIV. About 560,000 Americans are infected resulting from sexual transmission.	No cure. Considered by many as the almost perfect killing machine.	A person may look and feel healthy for years, but will be infected and contagious for life.

202

Test Your Knowledge

1. Match the correct answers. Some may have more than one answer.

    A. Herpes   B. Hepatitis B   C. HPV   D. AIDS

    _____ 1. Can cause warts and cancer.
    _____ 2. Can cause painful blisters.
    _____ 3. Referred to by some as the perfect
              killing machine.
    _____ 4. Can cause cancer of the liver.
    _____ 5. Cannot be cured.
    _____ 6. Can cause death.

2. Which STDs discussed in this chapter concern you the most? Why?

    _____

    _____

    _____

    _____

3. Using your own words, describe the effects of the human papilloma virus (HPV).

    _____

    _____

    _____

    _____

4.	Would it be difficult to have *SENSATIONAL SEX* if you or your partner had a viral STD? Explain.

_____

_____

_____

_____

5.	Look back over Lori's List. Write down any new information you feel Lori should consider about incurable STDs.

Family Discussion

1.	Check the answers to the workbook questions.

2.	How do you think you would feel if you had an incurable STD?

3.	Think back to the story told in the Herpes section where Kyle gave Mindy herpes.
	A.	Describe the impact the disease had on each of them.
	B.	Talk about when Mindy should tell future boyfriends that she has an incurable, highly contagious disease. Should she be honest and tell each new boyfriend when they first begin to date? Or should she wait until the relationship becomes serious and they are talking about marriage?
	C.	What about Kyle? When should he tell future girlfriends? Since he is asymptomatic, do you think he is as likely to tell future sexual partners about his STD? Explain.

4. Using the knowledge you gained from this chapter, explain how *CHOICES* about sex can lead to lifelong regrets.

5. Regarding the situation between Lori and Brian, if Brian assured Lori that he did not have an STD, would she then be safe? What if he assured her he *ALWAYS* practices "safe sex" by using a condom every time he has sex? Would she then be safe? Explain.

Additional Discussion

⇒ Parents, explain to your children what concerns you most about these incurable diseases.

⇒ What impact would an incurable STD have on the way a person feels about himself or herself?

⇒ Discuss why condoms do not always protect from STDs such as herpes and HPV.

⇒ If Lori does have sex with Brian, what kind of tests should she get afterwards? How long will she have to wait to find out if she may have contracted HIV from Brian?

⇒ Do you think having sex with Brian is worth the risk? At this point, what would you tell Lori?

References

[1]Fleming, Douglas. T., et al., *The New England Journal of Medicine*, October 16, 1997; 337(16) 1105.

[2]Ibid.

[3]Ibid., 1110.

[4]Centers for Disease Control and Prevention, Surveillance of hepatitis B in the U.S., website: cdc.gov/ncidad/diseases/hepatitis, June 3, 1998.

[5]Centers for Disease Control and Prevention, *Morbidity and Mortality Weekly Report,* 1991; 40:1-17.

[6]Kaiser Family Foundation, American Social Health Association, *Sexually Transmitted Diseases in American: How Many Cases and at What Cost?* Menlo Park, CA., December 1998.

[7]Ho, Gloria, Ph.D., et al., Natural History of Cervicovaginal Papillomavirus Infection in Young Women, *New England Journal of Medicine*, February 12, 1998; 338:7, 425.

[8]Cunningham, G.F. et al. (eds). *Williams Obstetrics* (20th ed.) Stanford, CT:Appleton and Lange, 1997;1332-1333.

[9]Institute of Medicine, *The Hidden Epidemic: Confronting Sexually Transmitted Diseases*, 1997; 43.

[10]Walboomers, J.M. et al. Human Papillomavirus is a Necessary Cause of Invasive Cervical Cancer Worldwide. *Journal of Pathology,* September 1999;189(1),12-19.

[11]National Institutes of Health. *Cervical Cancer. NIH Consensus Development Statement,* Online, April 1-3, 1996;43(1),1-30.

[12]Rodrigues, Barbra, "Health Officials Warn Teenage Girls of Cervical Cancer Risks," *The Dallas Morning News*, August 7, 1996; 29A.

[13]Institute of Medicine, *The Hidden Epidemic: Confronting Sexually Transmitted Diseases*, 1997; 31.

[14]Kaiser Family Foundation, American Social Health Association, *Sexually Transmitted Diseases in American: How Many Cases and at What Cost?* Menlo Park, CA., December 1998.

[15]Karon, J.M., et al., "Prevalence of HIV Infection in the United States, 1984 to 1992," *Journal of the American Medical Association*, July 1996; 276(2); 126-131.

[16]The Medical Institute for Sexual Health, *Sexual Health Today*, 1998; 75.

[17]Centers for Disease Control and Prevention, "Heterosexually Acquired AIDS - U.S.," *Morbidity and Mortality Weekly Report*, 1994; 43(9); 156-60.

[18]McIlhaney, Joe S., Jr. M.D., *Sex: What You Don't Know Can Kill You*, (Baker Books) 1997; 59-63.

[19]The National Institute of Health, Bethesda, MD, January 15, 1997.

Note to Parents

In this chapter, your child is going to learn that good *CHOICES* have good consequences and bad *CHOICES* can bring bad consequences. One result of poor sexual *CHOICES* is painful emotional scars. Emotional pain is hard to describe. It cannot be seen, only felt. That is why this chapter is filled with so many stories.

I have found younger teens often have a harder time understanding the concept of emotional scars than older teenagers. This is probably because of their lack of experience in serious relationships. All they know is what they see on television and the movies. Hollywood rarely shows lasting emotional scars. Let's face it, it is more exciting to sell hot, passionate sex than lifelong emotional scars.

One of the best things we can do as parents is to help our children learn that their actions have consequences. Learning this concept while they are young can eliminate a host of problems throughout their life. The following are a few ways you can teach your children about good and bad consequences.

- If they forget their lunch money or homework, don't rush to their aid. Going a day without lunch or taking an F on an assignment could leave a lasting impression.

- If your children get a traffic ticket, make them deal with all the necessary phone calls and arrangements, as well as paying for the ticket and the increased insurance rates.

- If they come home late with no reasonable excuse, don't overlook their irresponsible behavior. Make them pay a price, something that will cause them to work hard to be on time in the future.

- When your children make good *CHOICES*, make sure you praise them and reward them for such actions. As parents, we are often quick to criticize and slow to praise when we should be doing the reverse. Make the most of every opportunity to teach your children that their actions have consequences. In doing so, you may be protecting them from serious lifelong emotional scars.

A Tip from the Tool Box:

Praise your child more than you criticize him. All of us can only take so much criticism and then we shut down. Your child is no different. When you do need to criticize, make sure it is in the form of *constructive* criticism so he will be willing to learn from his mistakes. Treat your children with the same respect you would want your boss to treat you. Let your child overhear you bragging about him to a friend or relative. Praise his character, not just his achievements. The more you build him up, the more he will strive to improve.

Chapter 9

EMOTIONAL SCARS

When a close relationship comes to an end, there are often feelings of sorrow and emptiness. This pain can be greatly multiplied if the relationship was also sexual. Even if there was no pregnancy or STD, the emotional scars may linger for a lifetime.

This type of pain cannot be measured. Neither can it be cured by a simple round of antibiotics or removed by a surgical procedure. It's even difficult to describe. But it is very real. Psychologists tell us that having sex is the most intimate form of bonding known. So doesn't it make sense that when the sexual relationship is over, a person could have a sense of great loss, emptiness and painful memories? As you continue your search for *SENSATIONAL SEX*, you are going to want to learn how to make *CHOICES* which will protect you from a lifetime of emotional scars.

The regrets of sexual involvement were obvious when 500 high school students were surveyed. Sixty-two percent of the sexually experienced girls and 54 percent of all the teenagers who had experienced sex at least one time said they "should have waited."[1]

An even greater indication of this emotional distress comes from a survey conducted by the Indiana University School of Medicine. The survey reported that sexually active teenage girls are six times more likely to have attempted suicide than girls who are virgins.[2] If sexual intercourse had been a rich, rewarding experience for these girls, wouldn't they have fond memories when the relationship ended instead of suicidal thoughts?

While it is true that guys experience emotional pain, sometimes it seems that girls suffer the greater pain after a sexual encounter. Let me offer a possible explanation. You have probably heard that one of a man's greatest desires is sex. One of the greatest needs for a woman is love. When a sexual encounter is over, whether it lasted one night or several months, the man walks away having his sexual desires fulfilled while the woman is left feeling used. This was clearly demonstrated in the following true story.

A man told me that when he was in the ninth grade he had observed that girls really needed love. He also knew he really wanted sex. Therefore, he learned that if he could convince girls that he loved them, they would get what they needed and he would get what he wanted. He said he actually practiced saying the words "I love you" in the mirror each morning as he brushed his teeth. Over and over he would say those three little words, trying to sound sincere. With practice, he became very convincing. When he put his plan into action he was amazed at how well his scheme worked.

He said throughout high school and college he went from girl to girl expressing his love for each of them. In return they would give themselves to him completely. From his perspective, this was perfect. After all, everyone was getting what they wanted. Unfortunately, he said he never took the time to look back at his victims after each break-up. He said it wasn't until years later that he realized he had left these young women with serious emotional pain as they realized they had been used. You see, when the relationship ended he walked away having gotten what he wanted – sex. But not one of those young ladies got what she needed – love. Hearing the words "I love you" is not the same as being loved.

Building Memories

Throughout your life you will build memories. No doubt you have many fond memories of special events which will be with you the rest of your life – family vacations, hitting a home run, making the drill team, receiving a special award.

Your mind is like a photograph album filled with snapshots of memorable events. But unlike a photo album, you cannot choose to destroy the unpleasant pictures in your mind. The memories are etched deep within your brain with no delete button. Without warning, a fragrance or a song might suddenly spark a memory. It might be a fond memory which brings a smile to your face or a painful memory causing anguish.

Since sex is the most intimate form of bonding, your brain will automatically store vivid memories of this event. If the relationship ends, those memories stored deep within your brain can be replayed over and over whether you welcome them or not.

A woman told me of her personal experience with emotional scars. Before she met her husband she had a brief affair with her boss. She said the guy was a real jerk, but rumor had it that he was great at sex! Curiosity got the best of her and she gave in when he started making passes. There were no passionate words of love and commitment spoken between them. They both knew this was just about sex. She learned very quickly that the rumors were correct. Although he was a real jerk, he was very good at sex. The exciting fling didn't last long. When it was over, she experienced no serious pain or regrets. After all, it was just for fun.

The problems didn't come until a few years later after she was married. Although she is now deeply in love with her husband, she said he is not nearly as good at sex as her boss was. She despises the memories which flash through her mind at the most inopportune times. Painfully she confided, "If only I could erase each and every thought of that short-lived fling from my mind. How unfair to compare such a wonderfully devoted man to such a jerk. If only I had saved myself for my husband, I wouldn't be comparing the man I love with a man I despise."

Advantages of One Lifetime Partner

The sexual relationship Chuck and I experienced before we were married produced a great deal of emotional baggage. You see, sex before marriage can plant doubts and lack of trust. Doubts and distrust can weaken or destroy a relationship. Chuck and I had to work through our emotional baggage for years. However, one advantage we did experience was the fact that we have remained mutually monogamous throughout our entire lives. In other words, we have *never* had a sexual relationship with anyone except each other. As a result, we have NEVER had to deal with painful memories of past lovers.

For all I know, I am married to the world's greatest lover! I think it's great that Chuck has never compared me to his previous lovers, because there weren't any. There is so much freedom when ALL the snapshots in your mind are of your lifelong companion.

> Having only one lifetime partner
> guards the mind from painful memories!

What Goes Around Comes Around

All the *CHOICES* you make in life have consequences. Good *CHOICES* have good consequences; bad *CHOICES* have bad consequences. Those consequences may remain with you throughout your life. Recently, after finishing an adult seminar, two people told me their personal stories which illustrate the concept of *CHOICES* and consequences. Listen to both stories and compare.

A woman told me she dated a wonderful guy named Scott all through high school and into college. She was convinced she would take his name someday and be his wife. Despite their intense sexual desires, they were both committed to sexual abstinence until marriage.

As she continued with her story, she laughed and said, "You know, I did take Scott's last name and to this day he's one of my best friends, but he isn't my husband. He's my brother-in-law. That's right. I married Scott's brother."

"The great thing is," she continued, "my husband and Scott are not only brothers, they are best friends. Our families go on vacations and do things together all the time. But I can't imagine that being the case if Scott and I had shared a hot and heavy sexual relationship while we were dating. The commitment we made to sexual abstinence years ago gives us freedom to be the best of friends today."

Now compare the freedom she experiences to the other story. A man told me he has never returned to his high school or college reunions. He said, "I just can't face the girls of my past. I knew I was using them back then, and they know it now. Besides, there is no way I would introduce my wife to those women. She knows about my past, but I'm not about to let her put names and faces together."

Good *CHOICES* have good consequences; bad *CHOICES* have bad consequences. Either way, you will live with the consequences the rest of your life.

Teens Speak Out

The personal stories I have heard after speaking to tens of thousands of adults and teenagers are endless. Sex is a very personal subject and people of all ages have personal comments.

The most common response I get from adults is: "I never faced a pregnancy, I never got a sexually transmitted disease, but the emotional scars continue to tear me apart."

Unfortunately, I have comments from hundreds of students which reflect tremendous regret, pain, and sorrow. A girl in high school wrote, "The part you said about emotional scars is true. They never heal. It is one of the worst pains you could ever have."

Another girl wrote, "People do not know the pain that you go through after the first time and then you break up. It feels like someone is ripping your heart open and taking half of it out. Will this pain ever go away?"

A young man at a high school approached me at the end of a program and sadly said, "The stuff you said about emotional pain is real. I had a girlfriend, and I really loved her. We had sex and then she dumped me. The pain just doesn't stop."

Unfortunately, he is right. For many people the pain doesn't go away. They simply have to learn to live with it.

Protection from Emotional Scars

Although there is protection to reduce the chances of pregnancies and STDs, there is *absolutely nothing* to protect your heart from emotional scars. Only those who make the *CHOICE* to postpone sex until marriage are free from the painful memories and regrets of premarital sex.

At this time complete **Workbook Chapter 9** beginning on the following page.

Looking Inside

1. Think back in your life. Have you ever had someone make fun of you? You know, you're too skinny, fat, short, tall, etc. Or perhaps they made fun of your name or your clothes. Or . . . The list could go on and on. Almost everyone has had this experience sometime in his or her life. When you think about this experience can you still feel the hurt, the pain, maybe even the anger? I'll bet you can remember almost everything about it including who did it, where you were, the time of day, and exactly how you felt. Write down what you can remember.

    _____

    _____

    _____

    _____

2. The human mind is an amazingly complex system which records endless details about events. But remember, these were only words. If you have sex with someone, which is the most intimate form of bonding for humans, and then you break up, do you think painful emotional scars might result? Would these emotional scars be less painful than the pain you felt when someone hurt you with words, or would they be worse? Explain.

    _____

    _____

    _____

    _____

3. Have you ever done something you knew was bad, but nobody ever caught you? Perhaps it now looks like you got away with it. Do memories of the event ever flash through your mind? Are they good memories or do they make you feel sad? Did you really get away with it?

    _____

    _____

    _____

    _____

4. What is the only guaranteed protection from painful memories and regrets of premarital sex?

    _____

    _____

    _____

    _____

5. Look back over Lori's List. Is there anything you want to discuss with Lori regarding emotional scars?

Family Discussion

Perhaps you have heard people say sex is no big deal. As a family, read the following situation which comes from Pat Socia, national speaker and author. Then determine if you think sex is a big deal.

At the conclusion of a school assembly, a high school football player told Pat his story. He was visibly distraught as his voice shook and his eyes filled with tears. He said he had been in a serious relationship with his first and only love. She was also the only girl he had ever had sex with, and he planned to marry her someday. But just three days earlier he had learned that she had had sex with several of his teammates. He was going out of his mind at the thought of other guys touching her body and having sex with her.

(Pat Socia, *Weaving Character into Sex Education*, 1998, 27.)

Now discuss the following questions as you determine if sex is a big deal.

A. How would this young man feel if his girlfriend had simply talked to his teammates instead of having sex with them? Would he be this upset?

B. Would he have been this upset if she had eaten lunch with the teammates?

C. How would he have felt if she had danced with the other guys? Does this compare to having sex with them?

D. How long will it take for him to get over this pain? What long-term effects might this have on this young man?

E. Are the *CHOICES* a person makes about sex a big deal?

Additional Discussion

⇒ Do you think girls have more problems with emotional scars than guys? Explain.

⇒ How do guys and girls differ in the way they deal with emotional pain?

⇒ Compare the story in this chapter about the 9th grade boy who learned to say, "I love you" to the story about the woman who married her boyfriend's brother.

    A. How did the women differ in these two stories?

    B. How did the men differ?

    C. What long-term consequences did their *CHOICES* have on each of their lives?

    D. Do you hope your future spouse is living like the people in the story of the 9th grade boy or the story of the woman who married her boyfriend's brother? Explain.

⇒ How often do you see emotional scars on television and movies? When you do see it, how long does the pain usually last? Is this the same as real life?

References

[1]SIECUS and Roper Starch Organization, "Teens Talk about Sex: Adolescent Sexuality in the '90s," April 11, 1995; 25.

[2]Orr, D.P., et al., "Premature Sexual Activity as an Indicator of Psychosocial Risk," *Pediatrics*, February 1991; 87(2):141-147.

Note to Parents

This past week a fifty-year-old woman told me she was sexually abused on a regular basis by an uncle when she was a young girl. She said she knew she didn't like what was happening to her, but she had no idea what to do about it. Unfortunately, sexual abuse is very common today. One in three girls and one in six boys may experience at least one sexually abusive episode by the time they become adults.[1]

A Rhode Island Rape Center study of 1,700 sixth and ninth graders found that 65 percent of boys and 57 percent of girls believed it was acceptable for a male to force a female to have sex if the couple had been dating for six months.[2] With proper education and warning, some of these horrible ordeals might be avoided.

Sexual abuse is a sensitive subject. Therefore, you should carefully watch the reaction of your children. It is possible they have been abused without your knowledge. Watch carefully for any signs of withdrawal or uncomfortable reactions. Victims of abuse often feel scared, guilty, or even responsible for the abuse. You need to be prepared to respond with gentleness, patience, and love. If your child has been abused, you should consult with a professional counselor who has experience in working with sexual abuse victims.

Talking about sexual abuse and rape can be uncomfortable even for those who have never experienced such a terrible ordeal. However, it is important that you discuss this chapter with your child. Those who understand what sexual abuse is will be better prepared to know how to respond if they are ever placed in that situation.

A Tip from the Tool Box:

Give your child lots of love – everyday. Reports of sexual abuse have caused many parents to hesitate when it comes to physical contact with their children. However, young people need *healthy* touching. If they don't get it from you, they will look elsewhere. Hug your children, give them a nudge on the shoulder or a gentle pat on the back. Say the words, "I love you" and "I'm so proud of you" on a regular basis. Hide a note in their book bag or under their pillow reminding them about how special they are to you.

[1] Guidry, H.M., "Childhood Sexual Abuse: Role of the Family Physician," *American Family Physicians,* 1995; 51:407-14.
[2] Stodghill, Ron, "Where'd You Learn That?" *Time,* 6/15/98.

Chapter *10*

SEXUAL ABUSE AND RAPE

Abuse of any kind is extremely painful. Verbal abuse can be in the form of yelling and screaming or soft sarcasm. Physical abuse may include hitting or slapping. It can cause bruises, cuts, and broken bones. Both verbal and physical abuse can produce a great deal of emotional pain.

Sexual abuse is another type of offense. It occurs when a person offends another sexually in any way. Sexual abuse may include touching the sexual area of an unwilling or unsuspecting person or having sexual intercourse with them.

Victims of sexual abuse are usually younger and smaller than the abuser. The abuser can be *a family member, a friend or a stranger*. Unfortunately, most sexual abuse comes from family members or friends, not strangers. An abuser may be a young person or someone as old as your parents or grandparents.

Sexual abuse is a tragedy and can lead to extremely serious emotional scars in the victim. Unfortunately, this type of abuse is very common today. In fact, one in three girls and one in six boys may experience at least one sexually abusive episode by the time they become adults.[1]

After I spoke to a church youth group, the teens divided into several small groups to discuss the problems of sexual pressure. I went from group to group to answer questions they might have. My heart broke as I approached a group of nine high school girls and realized three of them were saying they had been sexually abused. One was by a boyfriend, a date rape. One was by an uncle whom the girl had loved dearly. The other was by a stepbrother.

I left the church that night with a heavy heart. I ached for these young girls and wished I could take away their pain and memories.

221

Sexually Abused Boys

Girls are not the only victims of sexual abuse. Many boys and young men fall prey to sexual abuse as well. Recently, a man told me how he was abused in the 7th grade. He said he was walking home from school when his swim coach pulled up beside him in a truck and offered him a ride home. The boy eagerly went with him. The coach then asked him if he would like to stop at his house for some lemonade. Again the boy quickly accepted, knowing his parents would not object. Unfortunately, what started out as an innocent ride and a simple glass of lemonade turned into sexual abuse. It started with talking, then looking at pictures of nude bodies, and then came the touching.

Recently, Sheldon Kennedy of the Boston Bruins pro hockey team came forward to tell the world of the sexual abuse he experienced as a young person. Sheldon's abuser was not a stranger. It was his hockey coach. During the time this man was abusing Sheldon, he was also named as Man of the Year by *Inside Hockey* magazine for his coaching and his crusade against violence in the sport.[2]

It is terribly confusing for a young person whose sexual appetite is just emerging to have an adult make sexual advances. This confusion is compounded when the adult is someone placed high on a pedestal by everyone in the community or who is in a close relationship with the victim.

Coming forward took a great deal of courage on Sheldon's part. As a result, he has become a great role model for today's youth. Sexual abuse should not be a secret. Like Sheldon, abuse victims need to come forward and talk about their pain. According to Sheldon, coming forward and talking about this has been his best therapy.[3]

Virginity is Given – Not Taken

Your virginity is a priceless gift which can only be GIVEN AWAY one time. Therefore, it is important to understand that if you were sexually abused YOU DID NOT GIVE ANYTHING AWAY. You were violated. Perhaps it started when you were too young to understand what was happening, or maybe you were forced against your will. No matter what the situation was, I personally believe if you were sexually abused you still have your virginity to give away when you choose. If everyone else gets to choose when they will give this gift away and to whom they will give it, you should be able to do the same!

Damage of Abuse

Usually, the greatest problem of sexual abuse is the emotional damage caused by the abuse. Sadly, many victims of abuse feel unworthy of respect. Once violated, they often follow a path of self-destruction, allowing others to continue to use and abuse them. Their self-image is shattered after the confusing and traumatic experience. Victims of abuse cannot change what happened to them, but they can make the *CHOICE* not to let this destroy them. They can also refuse to let others continue to use and abuse them.

Working through sexual abuse all alone is extremely difficult. Ignoring the situation and pretending it didn't happen never makes it go away. There are professional counselors who are trained to work with victims of abuse. Coming forward and talking about this, as Sheldon Kennedy did, is a major step toward healing from sexual abuse.

Beware of Sexual Abusers

You need to know that no one has the right to touch the private parts of your body. Naturally, there may be occasions when a physical examination is necessary by a doctor, but no family member, friend, or stranger has the right to do this.

Most coaches, youth leaders, parents and family members are NOT sexual abusers. But if you ever feel uneasy about or suspicious of a person, get away from them! If someone:

- tries to have a conversation with you about sexual matters
- wants to show you pictures or videos with sexual content
- wants to take seductive pictures or videos of you
- touches you inappropriately
- wants to have sexual intercourse with you

get out of there quickly and then tell your parents or another trusted adult.

223

A dead giveaway of a sexual abuser is that he or she will usually tell you this is to be a secret between the two of you. They may even threaten you or someone you love with harm if you tell anyone. That is all the more reason to tell someone.

If a person has sexually abused you (or has tried to), it is *very* likely that he or she is also abusing others. By reporting the situation you may save many others from serious problems.

Remember, child molesters and rapists may appear to be warm and charming. They may be admired by others and may have received various awards and honors. But behind the mask of kindness and greatness is a very disturbed person.

Our society desperately needs a healthy respect for sex. We need to understand that sex is very good and enjoyable under certain conditions, but outside those parameters sex can hurt deeply and be very destructive.

> Your body is very special, and no one
> has the right to touch you inappropriately

Rape

Rape is the fastest growing violent crime in America.[4] When a person is forced to have sex against his or her will, that is called rape. Rape is usually not so much about sex as it is about control and power. Rapes take place in homes, cars, schools, parks and alleys. A rapist may be a total stranger, someone you know, or even the person you are dating. Using common sense may help prevent some rapes. A few suggestions are:

- Avoid alcohol and drugs. You need to stay in control, not lose control.
- Avoid seductive clothes.
- Avoid seductive body language.
- Avoid walking alone at night. Even parking lots can be dangerous.
- Avoid going into an empty house, apartment, or building with people you do not know well.

- Avoid driving alone at night in unfamiliar areas, and keep your car doors locked.
- Avoid leaving a party with a stranger or getting a ride with a stranger.
- Avoid opening your door to a stranger, especially if you are home alone.

Unfortunately, many rapes cannot be prevented. A person can do everything right and still be brutally raped. But the old adage, "Better safe than sorry" may help prevent many attacks.

WARNING: No Means No

Guys must realize that when a girl says, "No," that is exactly what she means. A guy may think a girl is interested in having sex by the way she dresses or comes on to him. From his perspective her actions are saying, "I want to have sex with you." From her perspective, however, she may just be flirting with him and teasing him. While the game may be fun at first, she may suddenly realize he is moving too fast or going farther than she intended. It may also be possible she simply changed her mind. She might start struggling with him and telling him to stop.

At this point he may be so sexually aroused that he begins to think, "She doesn't really want me to stop. This is still part of the game she's playing. She's saying 'No' but she really wants it."

It doesn't matter how seductively a girl is dressed. It doesn't matter whether she said she wanted to have sex earlier. It doesn't matter whether you've had sex with her several times before. If at anytime she says, "NO" or "STOP," you had better stop dead in your tracks or you could be behind bars for a long time. Rape is always wrong. No one should ever be forced to have sex against their will.

What to Do

If you are ever a victim of rape, you should *immediately* call the police. Do NOT change your clothes or take a shower or bath. Try to remember as many details as possible to tell the police, such as the type of car, license number, race of the assailant, age, weight, height, hair color, clothing, unusual marks, tattoos, scars, rings, etc.

Rape can be extremely painful both physically and emotionally. Prosecuting the person who attacked you may not take your pain away, but it may stop the person from attacking other innocent victims.

At this time complete **Workbook Chapter 10** beginning on the following page.

Be on Your Guard

1. Sexual abusers can be either a

   A._____

   B._____

   C._____

2. One out of every _____ girls are sexually abused.

3. One out of every _____ boys are sexually abused.

4. Look back over the section "Beware of Sexual Abusers" and list five things which could be warning signs of a sexual abuser.

   A._____

   B._____

   C._____

   D. _____

   E. _____

5. Why do you think a sexual abuser would want you to keep the situation a secret?

   _____

   _____

6. Let's say a man who lived on your block invited you into his house. Then after you were inside he started talking about sex or wanting to show you some pictures and videos of people having sex. What two things should you do?

A._____

B._____

7. If a person is raped, that person should immediately _____ and should not change _____, take a _____, or _____. It is also important to remember _____.

8. Go to Lori's List and add any concerns she should consider about rape.

Family Discussion

1. Check your answers in the back of this book.

2. If a couple has been dating for several months and the guy has bought the girl several nice gifts and taken her out to some expensive places, is it okay for him to force her to have sex? Explain.

3. What if you found out one of your best friends had just been sexually abused by her uncle? What do you think she would be feeling? What concerns would you have about her? What advice would you give her?

4. Why is it important to tell an adult about sexual abuse or attempted sexual abuse?

Additional Discussion

⇒ The following is a story about two teenagers who were looking for fun on a Friday night, but something went wrong. Read the story and then discuss it together.

Julie was fifteen, a freshman in high school. She was also a virgin. One Friday night she attended a party where she consumed a couple of beers. She had never done much drinking and was amazed at how relaxed the two drinks made her feel. Then it happened. Jeff walked in the door. Julie knew who he was – everyone knew who he was – but he had no idea who she was. After all, Jeff was a senior and the quarterback of the football team; she was just a freshman. Julie amazed herself by walking right up to Jeff and asking him to dance. As they danced she amazed herself again by passionately kissing him, not once, but several times. This was not like Julie. She had always been fairly shy and reserved, but evidently a few beers changed all that.

After a few dances, Jeff suggested they leave and go to another party which wasn't so crowded and loud. Julie was thrilled to walk out with Jeff in front of all her friends. The two of them got in Jeff's car and drove to an apartment complex. When they walked inside, Julie immediately noticed there were no voices or music. Jeff shut the door. Then he shoved Julie against the wall and raped her.

Julie pressed charges, and Jeff was arrested for rape. Their friends at the party ended up being the witnesses in the trial. Everyone at the party saw Julie take a few drinks that night. Her friends testified, under oath, that she wasn't quite herself. They said it was Julie who approached Jeff at the party and asked him to dance. It was also Julie who initiated the passionate kissing. Then they all saw Julie willingly leave the party with Jeff. But no one saw what happened in the apartment. It was Julie's word against Jeff's.

Jeff swore that Julie wanted to have sex with him. He said he knew what she was really wanting as soon as she asked him to dance. She confirmed her intentions by passionately kissing him while they were dancing. Jeff said he just gave her what she wanted.

Julie said she was just having fun that night and the thought of having sex had never crossed her mind. She said that just because she asked Jeff to dance and kissed him a couple of times did not mean she wanted to have sex with him. Yes, she left the party with him, but he told her they were going to another party. He lied to her. She said she would have never gone to the apartment with him if she had known they would be all alone. She said when he started raping her she begged him to stop. She cried for help, but there was no one there to hear her cries.

You Be The Judge . . .

1. As a family, decide if you think Jeff was guilty of rape. Discuss what could happen if a jury convicted Jeff of rape.

2. Julie made several *CHOICES* that night which ended up being mistakes. Discuss her mistakes.

3. What long-term physical and emotional consequences may Julie have to deal with as a result of the *CHOICES* she made?

4. Did the alcohol Julie consumed at the party play a part in this? Explain.

5. How would self-control, self-respect, and self-discipline have made a difference for Julie? How would self-control, self-respect, and self-discipline have made a difference for Jeff?

References

[1]Guidry, H.M., "Childhood Sexual Abuse: Role of the Family Physician." *American Family Physician*, 1995; 51:407-414.

[2]McCallum, Jack, "Betrayed Trust," *Sports Illustrated*, January 13, 1997; 86(1):15-16.

[3]Ibid.

[4]Dallas Police Department, *Rape - Suggestion for Self Protection*, 1998.

Chapter 11
Lack of Self Control

Note to Parents

In this chapter your children will learn the importance of self-control. They will consider the difference between people who learn to control their sexual desires and those who do not.

During the discussion time your children will be asked to share their strongest character traits. Don't be surprised if your children have a difficult time seeing their own strengths. Teenagers can be very hard on themselves. Take this opportunity to build your child's self-esteem by sharing a list of his or her attributes.

During the Additional Discussion you will be given the opportunity to suggest that your child select an accountability partner. Give this concept some serious consideration. It could prove to be very helpful to your child. This person can become your child's mentor and role model, a person who can help guide, direct, and encourage your child to strive for excellence. No doubt, you are already fulfilling this role. However, today's youth cannot have too many positive role models taking a genuine interest in their lives. Perhaps the two of them could make a one-year commitment to go out for dinner or ice cream every few weeks and just talk. This person should be *at least* five years older than your child, fun to be around, and capable of challenging your child to strive for excellence.

A Tip from the Tool Box:

> Teach your children what good, healthy dating is all about by taking them out for special times together. Dad, call your daughter on the phone and ask her for a date. Treat her with the dignity and respect you would expect from other young men. Mom, go to dinner with your son. Let him place the order for both of you. After the meal let him pay the check, leave the tip, and escort you back to the car. (Don't forget to give him the money before you leave home, since he probably doesn't have that kind of money from his allowance.) Remember, the pregnancy rate is lower among young people who share activities with their parents.

Chapter 11

LACK OF SELF CONTROL

Having sexual desires is very normal and natural, but as humans we are capable of controlling these urges. Just as you learned to control the natural urge to go to the bathroom around the age of two, now you can learn to control the natural urge to have sex.

If someone in your school went around wetting his pants, you would probably think that person is really lacking self control. A person who cannot control their sexual urges is also seriously lacking self control. As you continue your search for *SENSATIONAL SEX*, you need to understand the importance of gaining control of your sexual desires. Let me explain.

Let's say Johnny and Susie begin dating. They fall in love and have sex. Eventually they get married. On their wedding day there will probably be a great sense of relief as they realize they were indeed one of the lucky ones! No pregnancy. No STDs. And here they are about to get married.

However, they might be facing problems they never considered. You see, while they were dating they never developed the discipline of self control. This part of their character was never strengthened. So, why should we suppose that just because they have placed rings on their fingers, said a few vows, and signed a piece of paper that they will suddenly be capable of practicing self control?

What happens six months or ten years down the road when Johnny goes off to work and some gorgeous young woman starts coming on to him? He didn't say no to sexual desires before marriage. Are we sure he can do it now?

Or let's say Johnny starts working long hours and Susie begins feeling neglected and less desirable. What would happen if a gorgeous hunk came into her life and began telling her how beautiful she is? Do you think she will be able to say no to these sexual desires when this character trait was never developed?

The Benefits of Self Control

Let's compare this scenario to the real life story of my friends, Mark and Pat. They had a serious relationship for three years before they got married. During that time Mark never attempted to touch Pat. Oh sure, he kissed her, held her hand and put his arm around her, but he never touched her intimately. Now, keep in mind, Mark is no geek. He is a good-looking body builder who loves rock climbing.

Stop and think a moment about their honeymoon. No pregnancy. No STDs. No past memories of former lovers. For three years the passion has built. And now, after public vows and promises, they privately give themselves to each other for the first time. WOW! That's romantic . . . and a lot of fun!

By the way, Pat has shared with me that Mark's muscles and good looks were not what impressed her the most when they were dating. It was his strong character, self discipline and self control that really impressed her.

Pat and Mark have now been married for several years. Mark is still a good-looking body builder. He is also a very successful businessman who travels regularly throughout the United States and Europe. But Pat never worries about her husband being unfaithful while he is out of town. She knows the strong character which controlled his sexual appetite during their three years of dating will continue to provide the discipline to wait a week or two when he is away from home.

Self Control is a Sign of Strength

Chain Reaction

When a person has the strength to control their sexual desires, a natural chain reaction occurs. The self control, self respect, and self discipline required to control the human sex drive will begin to spill over into all areas of that person's life. Although difficult to achieve, these character qualities help build a strong foundation which will empower a person to meet other difficult challenges throughout life.

A natural chain reaction will also occur for those whose character foundation is weak. This weakness can unleash a chain reaction which can come back to haunt a person throughout life. Research has shown:

Teenage boys who have had sex are:
- 6 times more likely to drink alcohol than virgin teenage boys
- 4 times more likely to smoke cigarettes
- 5 times more likely to smoke marijuana
- 4 times more likely to use other drugs
- 7 times more likely to consider dropping out of school
- 3 times more likely to run away from home
- 4 times more likely to be arrested by the police
- 7 times more likely to be suspended from school than virgin teenage boys

Teenage girls who have had sex are:
- 6 times more likely to drink alcohol than virgin teenage girls
- 7 times more likely to smoke cigarettes
- 10 times more likely to smoke marijuana
- 4 times more likely to use other drugs
- 4 times more likely to consider dropping out of school
- 18 times more likely to run away from home
- 9 times more likely to be arrested by the police
- 5 times more likely to be suspended from school
- 6 times more likely to attempt suicide than virgin teenage girls[1]

Facing Life's Problems

One of the few guarantees you have in life is that you WILL face problems. There is no escape. Some problems will be small and insignificant, but unfortunately some will be devastating and tragic. What would happen if you had a big business deal that went bad and you were suddenly facing bankruptcy? What if one of your children was born with a serious birth defect? Suppose you were diagnosed with cancer. What type of person would you want standing by your side in the midst of tragic situations such as these? Would it help to know that your lifelong partner has a track record of strength and discipline in the midst of problems and pressure?

To control the powerful sex drive a person must be:

strong
focused
motivated
determined
self confident
highly disciplined
respectful of others
able to withstand ridicule
able to withstand temptation
able to withstand peer pressure
concerned for others' well being

Is this the kind of person you would like to be? Is this the kind of person with whom you would like to spend your life?

> You can learn to control your sex drive
> or your sex drive can control you.

The *CHOICES* you make can lead to lifelong success or a lifetime of regret.

Now complete **Workbook Chapter 11** beginning on the following page.

Gaining Control

1. Self control is an important character trait. Without it there can be serious problems later in life. Look back at the first story in this chapter about Johnny and Susie. Where did they lack self control?

    _____

2. Compare the story of Johnny and Susie to the next story of Mark and Pat. Which couple do you think would be more likely to remain faithful to each other throughout their years of marriage? Explain your answer.

    _____

    _____

3. Put a √ by each phrase which describes the type of person you would like to date.

_____	Drinks alcohol
_____	Smokes cigarettes
_____	Uses drugs
_____	Hangs out with drug users
_____	High school drop out
_____	Has a police record
_____	Suspended from school
_____	Suicidal

4. How many √'s did you put down on question number 3?

    _____

5. Does that list describe the type of person you want to date or marry?   Yes   No

6.   Does it describe the type of person you want to become?
        Yes   No

7.   In this chapter, you were given the results of a national study which compared teenagers who have had sex with those who have not had sex. The findings of that study showed that teens who have had sex are far more likely to do the things listed in number 3 than those who have not had sex. With all this in mind, do you want to date people who are sexually active or would you rather date people who have learned to control their sex drive? Explain your answer.

        _____

        _____

        _____

        _____

8.   Go back to Lori's List in Workbook Chapter 2 and write down any new ideas which Lori should consider about self control.

Family Discussion

1.   When a person learns to control their sex drive, a natural chain reaction will occur. Describe this chain reaction.

2.   Describe what the chain reaction might be if the sex drive is not brought under control. (You might want to refer back to the comparison in this chapter of teens who have had sex with those who have not.)

3.   How do others see you? If you applied for a job and the business contacted your references to check on your character,

what would others say about you? "He/she is (dependable, honest, loyal, courteous, self-confident, trustworthy, well respected, respectful of others, determined, high achiever, etc.)."

4. Discuss the differences between the dating relationship of a couple who is in control of their sexual desires versus a couple who is controlled by their sexual desires.
    *   What would each couple do on their dates?
    *   Where would they go and what would they hope to accomplish on their dates?

5. Think of friends and relatives who have faced some tragic, difficult issues. Can you see some examples of character strength or weakness being displayed during these difficult times? In these situations were they acting as positive role models?

Additional Discussion

⇒ Every successful professional athlete has a coach guiding, directing and encouraging them to strive for excellence. How about selecting an adult whom you admire and asking them to become your personal coach or accountability partner? No doubt your parents care a great deal about you, but it might be nice to have an accountability partner who isn't quite so close to home. Perhaps this could be a neighbor, an aunt or uncle, or maybe someone from your church or synagogue. Perhaps the two of you could meet together every couple of weeks and have dinner or go out for ice cream and just talk. The person should:

1. Know your family well.
2. Be at least five years older than you.
3. Be someone you respect and see as a great role model.

Make a list of possible accountability partners.

1. _____

2. _____

3. _____

References

[1]Orr, D.P., et al., "Premature Sexual Activity as an Indicator of Psychosocial Risk," *Pediatrics*, February 1991; 87(2):141-147.

The Search for Perfect Protection

Note to Parents

Your children are not going to make *CHOICES* that lead to lifelong success about sex unless they have knowledge and understanding about contraceptives. I have spoken to thousands of students from 5th to 12th grade across the country. When I ask them, "How can you *guarantee* you will not face a pregnancy or get an STD?" the usual answer is, "USE A CONDOM!" How sad when well-educated students believe a condom will *guarantee* freedom from pregnancies and STDs.

Pat Socia has phrased it best. She stated, "When a condom is used consistently and correctly, it will reduce some of the risk of some of the diseases some of the time." That's a long way from being a *guaranteed* solution!

This chapter will provide your children with accurate information about the leading forms of contraceptives. However, the chapter provides "typical" or "real life" results as opposed to findings from laboratories, which is what young people often hear about. This chapter clearly teaches that while condoms, pills, injections and implants might reduce some of the risk some of the time, abstinence is the only *guaranteed* plan of protection that works 100 percent of the time.

Our country has spent billions of taxpayers' dollars over the past 25 years to teach our children that "Abstinence is best, *but* if you are going to do it anyway, then make sure you use condoms consistently and correctly." The problem is, this is a mixed message. It is like telling a four year old, "I do not want you having any snacks before dinner, *but* if you feel you just have to eat something, make sure you only have one piece of candy." Will that child eat the candy before his dinner? Of course he will. Why shouldn't he? He was given permission.

Here's another way of looking at this: Let's say the issue was shoplifting instead of sexual activity. Shoplifting is something many teenagers are trying today. It isn't that they need the objects being taken. It's more like a game they are playing.

Let's say you suspected your child was involved in this game and felt it was time for a direct talk. You might explain to your child that some things in life are just wrong, and stealing falls into that category. As you continue, you might say that shoplifting could go on your child's permanent record or perhaps result in a jail sentence. You would probably go so far as to say, "I *do not* want you involved in any type of shoplifting."

But could you imagine following that statement by saying, "*But,* if you feel you just have to shoplift, then let me give you a few ideas on how to do it safely." And then you give three or four clever tips on how to steal without being caught.

While this may sound absurd, there is little difference in teaching the importance of sexual abstinence as your value and then saying, "*But,* if you are going to have sex anyway, then let me teach you how to do it safely." Remember, there is no such thing as safe sex. The best you can do is to help your child reduce *some* of the risk of *some* of the problems *some* of the time. Is that what you want for your children?

Teachers and parents are giving mixed messages when they say, "It would be best if you did not have sex, *but* if you do, make sure you use a condom." Whether they realize it or not, that mixed message is giving permission for the child to have sex. Today's youth do not need mixed messages. They need absolutes. This has been confirmed by a study released by the U.S. government which states that sexual activity among teenagers goes down when parents tell their children they disapprove of them having sex and using contraceptives.[1]

What a difference it makes when parents tell their children, "I love you and because of that love I DO NOT want your to have sex until you get married! I know abstinence won't be easy, but I believe you can succeed!"

A Tip from the Tool Box:

Help your children to dress and look their age. A national government study found that young people who perceive themselves as looking older than their same-age peers have sexual intercourse at a younger age. They are also more likely to use cigarettes, alcohol, and marijuana. Once in high school, they are more likely to experience emotional distress or to think about or attempt suicide than those who perceive themselves as looking age-appropriate.[2]

---

[1] Resnick, Michael, D., Ph.D., et al., "Protecting Adolescents from Harm: Findings from the National Longitudinal Study on Adolescent Health," *Journal of the American Medical Association,* 9/10/97.
[2]Ibid.

Chapter 12

THE SEARCH FOR THE
PERFECT PROTECTION

You have probably figured out that a key element to *SENSATIONAL SEX* is preventing the bad and enjoying the good. Now that you understand how serious the bad can be, you need to figure out how to protect yourself from all of the problems.

The following chart shows the protection rate for the leading methods of contraceptives. The rates provided are real-life results as opposed to laboratory testing. For example, according to laboratory tests, condoms work 98% of the time to prevent pregnancy. But in real life, among real people using condoms in the heat of passion, condoms work approximately 84% of the time. Since you live in the real world, the following real life numbers should prove helpful in selecting your form of protection.

Method	Protection Rate For			
	Pregnancy	HIV	HPV	Emotional Scars
Withdrawal	76%	None	None	None
Condom	84%	57% to 90%	Almost None	None
Birth Control Pills	94%	None	None	None
Depo-Provera	99%	None	None	None
Norplant	99%	None	None	None
Abstinence	100%	100%	100%	100%

Note: Pregnancy Rates are based on a one-year average for women ages 15 to 44 and may vary with age.[1]

Methods of Protection

Withdrawal

When a man removes his penis from the woman's vagina before he ejaculates, this is called withdrawal. This is not an effective way to prevent pregnancy since small amounts of seminal fluid are released throughout sexual intercourse. These small drops contain thousands of sperm which can still produce a baby. (Remember, it only takes one sperm to fertilize the egg.) This method provides no protection from STDs or emotional scars.

The Condom

The condom is a thin balloon-like latex covering which fits snugly over a man's penis during sexual intercourse. Condoms can be bought over the counter and cost 10 to 12 dollars for a pack of 12. Condoms will not work unless they are fresh and stored properly to avoid extreme hot or cold temperatures. That means a man's wallet, a lady's purse, or a glove compartment of a car are not acceptable places to store a condom.

Although the condom will reduce the chance of pregnancy, it is not one of the more effective methods of birth control. A condom can, however, *reduce* (not eliminate) the spread of many STDs (including HIV) if it is used consistently and correctly *every time* a person has sex. You must understand, however, that the condom only protects the area it covers. Therefore the condom does NOT prevent the transmission of all STDs. For example:

Herpes – The New England Journal of Medicine recently stated that the condom gives "limited" protection from genital herpes because the virus can "occur on areas of the body not covered by condoms."[2]

HPV – The condom does little to prevent the spread of the human papilloma virus (HPV), the STD which can cause genital warts and cancer. This incurable STD can spread throughout the entire genital area including the buttocks, crease of the legs, inner thigh, and the male's scrotum. These areas are NOT covered by the condom. Skin to skin contact can spread this virus from one person to another.[3]

Those infected with HPV often have no visible signs or symptoms but are still highly contagious.

HIV – When the condom is used consistently and correctly every time a person has sex it will *reduce* (not eliminate) the risk of HIV. There have been several studies on the effectiveness of condoms against HIV. Three combined studies from Europe and Haiti show an effective rate of 90%.[4] Another study reported an effective rate of 69%.[5] A study from Brazil reported an effective rate of 57%.[6] When you do the math you realize condoms fail somewhere between 10 to 43 percent of the time in preventing AIDS. Is that safe enough for you?

Guidelines for Condom Use

Condoms must be used consistently and correctly *every time* a person has sex. The Centers for Disease Control and Prevention recommends the following five steps as guidelines for correct condom use:

1. Use a new condom with each act of intercourse.
2. Put on the condom as soon as erection occurs and before any sexual contact.
3. Hold the tip of the condom and unroll it onto the erect penis, leaving space at the end of the condom, yet ensuring that no air is trapped in the condom's tip.
4. Adequate lubrication is important but use only water-based lubricants such as glycerine or lubricating jellies. Oil-based lubricants, such as petroleum jelly, cold cream, lotion, or baby oil can weaken the condom.
5. Withdraw from the partner immediately after ejaculation, holding the condom firmly to keep it from slipping off.[7]

The Birth Control Pill

The Pill is an oral contraceptive taken by women which effectively reduces the risk of a pregnancy. To be effective, however, it should be taken *every day at the same time*. If a pill is missed, it reduces the protection rate. The pill often has side-effects, which may include irregular bleeding, weight gain and headaches.[8] The Pill costs approximately $240 a year and a prescription must be obtained from a physician.

The Pill provides no protection from sexually transmitted diseases or emotional scars.

Depo-Provera

Depo-Provera is an injection for women which prevents pregnancy for three months. This method is highly effective in preventing pregnancy. Side effects are irregular bleeding, weight gain, headaches, and possible dizziness. Adverse effects can last seven to eight months after the last shot.[9] It costs about $250 a year.

Depo-Provera provides no protection from sexually transmitted diseases or emotional scars.

Norplant

Norplant consists of six matchstick-size implants which are inserted under the skin of a woman's upper arm. These implants release protection from pregnancy for five years. This is a highly effective long-term form of birth control. However, Norplant is losing its popularity because of lawsuits. There are also complaints about complications in removing the implants. Side effects are irregular bleeding and weight gain.[10] The cost is approximately $120 a year.

Norplant provides no protection from sexually transmitted diseases or emotional scars.

Abstinence

Sexual abstinence is the decision to save sex until marriage. Those who have no sexual contact until marriage *never* worry about a pregnancy before marriage. There are no pills to take, shots or implants to deal with, and no failure rates to worry about. Abstinence works 100% of the time! Side effects are self control, self respect, and self discipline. These strong character traits tend to last a lifetime.

Two people who choose sexual abstinence until marriage and then remain faithfully committed to each other for a lifetime never worry about STDs. They will never have to bother with using condoms consistently and correctly every time they have sex. Nor will they ever need to remember the "Guidelines for Condom Use." After marriage they are free to have fun and enjoy their sexual intimacy anytime they choose with *no fear* of sexually transmitted diseases.

Sexual abstinence also eliminates the painful memories of past lovers. The condom, birth control pill, Depo-Provera, and Norplant do not protect against such emotional scars.

If a couple is ready for marriage and does not want to start a family immediately, they can consult with their physician, clergy, marriage counselor, parents and friends in considering the best form of birth control to prevent a pregnancy.

Selecting Your Method of Protection

As you consider your choice of protection, you need to decide:

> Do you want to *reduce* some of your risks
> or eliminate all of your risks?

As you consider your *CHOICES*, realize that sexual activity can be as dangerous as walking in a deadly explosive minefield. You must select one option:

1. Would you walk into that minefield with **no protection** at all? Those who have unprotected sex outside of marriage today have little chance of escaping serious to life-threatening injuries.

2. Would you walk confidently into a minefield if you had a bulletproof vest and a helmet on for protection? This protective gear can give **limited protection** in a minefield, but with one wrong step you could still lose a leg, or even worse, your life. In a similar way, even if you protect yourself with one or more forms of contraception, an STD could still invade your body, causing cancer, sterility or death.

3. If you avoided the minefield altogether, you would **eliminate ALL dangers and fears**. Couples who choose sexual abstinence until marriage do just that.

They never experience the fear and worries of pregnancies before marriage, STDs, and the trauma of emotional scars. Before marriage they are free to enjoy and grow in their relationship while avoiding all the life-threatening problems. After marriage, they can have fun and enjoy their sexual intimacy completely free from problems from their past.

So, what form of protection do you prefer:

No protection?
Limited protection?
Guaranteed protection?

It's your life. It's your decision. You must choose for yourself.

Now complete **Workbook Chapter 12** beginning on the following page.

Protecting Yourself

Think about the information you have learned about contraceptives.

1. Which method is the only guaranteed protection from pregnancy?

    _____

2. Which method is the only guaranteed protection from STDs?

    _____

3. Which method will best prepare you for a healthy marriage? Explain.

    _____

    _____

4. Which method do you hope your future spouse is using right now? Explain.

    _____

    _____

    _____

5. Which method are you going to choose? Explain.

    _____

    _____

    _____

Family Discussion

Read the following story together, then answer the questions:

When Amber was 15 her mother took her to a clinic and started her on birth control pills. Amber's mother was very protective and wanted to make sure Amber never dealt with an unplanned pregnancy. Although Amber had never had sex and didn't even have a boyfriend, she obediently took her pill before she went to bed each night.

Two months later Amber met Bret. He was 18 and a senior in high school. Within two weeks, they had sex. But there was nothing to worry about. Amber was on the pill. Three weeks later, Bret's old girlfriend came back on the scene. She was 17 and gorgeous. Bret quickly dumped Amber, and her heart was broken.

The next week Amber was at a party. She was still hurting deeply over the loss of Bret until Keith started talking to her. Keith was Bret's best friend. That night Amber and Keith had sex. But there wasn't anything to worry about. Amber was on the pill and Keith used a condom.

The next day Amber saw Keith at the mall with one of the cheerleaders from her school. When she walked up to him, he acted like he didn't even know who she was. Once again, Amber was deeply hurt. This time she went straight home and threw her birth control pills in the trash and vowed she was finished with boys.

Two days later, her doorbell rang. It was Keith. He said he was so sorry about the incident at the mall, and he really wanted to see her. Reluctantly, Amber agreed to go out with him. Keith apologized over and over. He told her he loved her and really needed her. That night Keith and Amber had sex. Although Keith didn't have any condoms, there was nothing to worry about because as soon as Amber got home she rummaged through the trash and got her pills. She quickly took all three pills at once. Does Amber have anything to worry about?

1. Use the information you learned in this chapter and discuss how "safe" Amber is from a pregnancy and STDs. Name at least three people who could have been involved in passing an STD to Amber.

2. Did the contraceptives protect her heart from emotional scars?

3. Did the pill improve Amber's popularity?

4. What did the pill do to her reputation?

5. Why do you suppose Bret's best friend decided to talk to Amber at the party?

6. Use your imagination and talk about how this story might end for Amber, Keith, and Bret.

7. When a guy hears that a girl is using birth control, he often sees her as an easy target for sex. In reality, he should be seeing red flags and be concerned. Explain why.

Additional Discussion

⇒ Television and movies often show romantic love scenes. However, they never seem to show condoms being used. Look back over the "Guidelines for Condom Use" and try to imagine these steps being followed in the midst of a hot passionate love scene in a movie. Why do you think Hollywood avoids condoms?

⇒ Which form of protection are you choosing? Explain. What form of protection do you hope your future spouse is using right now?

References

[1]Rubin, Rita, "News You Can Use – Birth Control Failure," (Source: The Alan Guttmacher Institute) *U.S. News and World Report*, March 3, 1997; 67.

[2]Fleming, Douglas. T., et al., *The New England Journal of Medicine*, October 16, 1997; 337(16): 1110.

[3]National Institutes of Health. *Cervical Cancer. NIH Consensus Development Statement,* Online, April 1-3, 1996;43(1),1-30.

[4]deVincenzi, I., "A Longitudinal Study of HIV Transmission by Heterosexual Partners," *The New England Journal of Medicine*, 1994; 331(6):341-346.
Saracco, Alberto, et al. "Man-to-Woman Sexual Transmission of HIV: Longitudinal Study of 343 Partners of Infected Men," *Journal of Acquired Immune Deficiency Syndromes*, 1993; 6(5): 497-502.

[5]Weller, Susan C., "A Meta-Analysis of Condom Effectiveness in Reducing Sexually Transmitted HIV," *Social Science Medicine*, 1993; 36(12):1635-1644. Weller's finding was cited in the Centers for Disease Control and Prevention, "Update: Barrier Protection Against HIV Infection and Other Sexually Transmitted Diseases," *Morbidity and Mortality Weekly Report*, August 6, 1993; 42(30).

[6]Guimaraes, M.D.C., et al., "HIV Infection Among Female Partners of Seropositive Men in Brazil," *American Journal of Epidemiology*, 1995; 142(5): 538-547.

[7]Centers for Disease Control and Prevention, HIV/AIDS Prevention, "Facts about Condoms and Their Use in Preventing HIV Infection and Other STDs," July 30, 1993.

[8]Earl, D.T. & David, D.J., "Depo-Provera: An Injectable Contraceptive," *American Family Physician*, March 1994; 49(4): 891.

[9]Ibid.

[10]Rubin, Rita, "News You Can Use: Birth Control Failure," *U.S. News and World Report*, March 3, 1997; 66-68.

BOOK TWO

SECTION THREE

WOW! I CAN SUCCEED!

How to prevent the bad
and enjoy the good!

Chapter 13

The Secret to SENSATIONAL SEX

Note to Parents

This is the chapter where commitments begin. Up until now your child has been gathering information. Now it is time to begin making decisions.

You might want to consider providing your child with a commitment card. It might be fun to create a card with your child. This series also provides a commitment card which is suitable for framing. Information about the Student Commitment Certificate and the Parent Commitment of Love Certificate is provided at the end of Chapter 2 in the first section of this book under Additional Available Items.

As stated earlier, a national study found that sexual activity among teenagers decreases when young people know their parents disapprove of teenage sexual activity. This same study reported that:

> Teenagers who take a pledge to remain a virgin
> until marriage are more likely to delay intercourse.[1]

Commitment cards are only beneficial for young people who have truly bought into the abstinence movement. A young person who signs a commitment card to please Mom and Dad is signing it for the wrong reason. When faced with the heat of passion, the purpose of that card will quickly vanish.

If you decide to offer your children a commitment card, do *not* pressure or make them feel obligated to sign the certificate; and do not use this as a means to measure success or failure. Some young people will buy into the concept of sexual abstinence, but they don't like the concept of signing certificates. That's okay! Other young people will eagerly sign it and want to frame it.

If your child has not bought into the concept of sexual abstinence, DO NOT consider yourself a failure. The mere fact that you are at the end of the series proves you have NOT failed. By this point you have successfully provided your child with valuable information and family values. Give your child time and keep providing unconditional love! Remember, you *cannot* make *CHOICES* for your child. You can only provide good information.

If your child signs the certificate, remind him or her that signing the certificate is easy. Living the lifestyle is not! These last three chapters will provide practical suggestions on how to succeed in this lifestyle.

A Tip from the Tool Box:

Help your children understand that abstinence and alcohol do not mix. In fact, alcohol and drugs are a major factor in sexual activity. Sixty percent of college girls who acquired STDs, including herpes and AIDS, were drunk at the time of the infection. And 90 percent of rapes that occurred on campus happened when alcohol was used by the victim, the perpetrator, or both.[2]

[1]Resnick, Michael. D, Ph.D., et al. "Protecting Adolescents from Harm: Findings from the National Longitudinal Study on Adolescent Health." *Journal of the American Medical Association,* 9/10/97.
[2] Center of Addiction and Substance Abuse (CASA), Columbia University, New York, 1994.

Chapter 13

THE SECRET TO
SENSATIONAL SEX

The only people who can enjoy a lifetime of *SENSATIONAL SEX* with NO FEAR of STDs are those who remain SEXUALLY ABSTINENT until marriage and then remain FAITHFUL to each other for life.

Condoms are not the secret. Pills, implants and injections are not the secret. Building the strong character traits of self control, self respect, and self discipline while waiting until marriage is the only way which *guarantees freedom* from the destructive problems associated with premarital sex. Perhaps that is why married couples have more fulfilling sex lives than single people.

That's right. While Hollywood may paint an exciting picture of the single lifestyle, in real life it is married couples who report being the "most physically pleased and emotionally satisfied" when it comes to sex.[1] According to a national study, physical and emotional satisfaction start to decline when people have more than one sexual partner.[2]

> Married couples have more fulfilling
> sex lives than single people!

Now that you have *knowledge* and *understanding* regarding the secret of *SENSATIONAL SEX*, you must decide what you will do with that knowledge. Will you make *CHOICES* that lead to lifelong success or will you take a chance and hope to escape a lifetime of regrets? The *CHOICE* is yours.

259

Is Abstinence Possible?

The message of sexual abstinence only began to strongly re-emerge in the U.S. in the past ten years. During this time, groups throughout the country started raising the standard for young people by encouraging the concept of sexual abstinence until marriage. Many adults laughed, saying teenagers could NEVER meet such high standards and would NEVER consider such a radical lifestyle.

But observe closely and you will notice the laughter has now stopped as teenagers throughout the country are taking a strong stand for sexual abstinence. The verdict is still out, but the early returns look promising!

> On May 1, 1997, the U.S. government
> announced the sexual activity rate
> among teenagers had dropped
> for the first time in 25 years![3]

> On September 18, 1998, the U.S. government
> announced that teen sexual activity rates
> have continued to drop and more than
> half of American high school students
> (males and females) are virgins![4]

An Impressive Role Model

Consider A.C. Green. He is a professional basketball player who has played with the L.A. Lakers, Phoenix Suns, Dallas Mavericks, and is now back with the Lakers. On November 20, 1997 he set the NBA record of playing in 907 consecutive games. He is a rich, successful basketball star. He is also a virgin . . . and PROUD of it!

That's right. A.C. Green has never had sex. Does he ever think about sex or desire sex? Sure he does! However, he made a *CHOICE* many years ago to develop the self control necessary to focus on his goals and save sex for marriage.[5]

Setting the record for the most consecutive games in the NBA did not come easy. It required a great deal of determination, dependability, discipline, and the ability to play despite painful injuries. The story in *Sports Illustrated* featuring A.C. was entitled, "Iron Man." Impressive title. Impressive man!

Understanding the Challenges

Postponing sex until marriage is more difficult today than ever before. For one reason, the onset of puberty, or sexual awakening, starts at a younger age. A hundred years ago the average age of puberty was 15 to 16. Today, it is around 11 to 13. To add to this problem, the average age of marriage is 27 for men and 25 for women.[6]

Do you see the problem? If you accept this challenge of sexual abstinence until marriage, that means on average you may wait 12 to 15 years from puberty to marriage. Wow! That's asking a lot.

What If It's Too Late?

It is NEVER too late to choose the best for your life! Obviously, you cannot undo what has already been done. But you can stop right now before additional damage is done.

Recently, a young man told me he and his girlfriend stopped having sex three years ago because of their commitment to abstinence. One young lady wrote me a note which said, "I heard you speak two years ago, and I have not had sex since because you made me think."

After speaking to 100 girls at a drill team camp, one of the instructors came up and told me her story. She said, "Marilyn, you spoke at my school four years ago when I was in the ninth grade. The day I heard this program I was dying inside. You see, I had already had sex with 3 different guys. As you spoke that day, I realized I had made a real mess of my life. I kept thinking, 'It's too late!' Then you began to talk about how it's never too late to choose the best for your life. I listened carefully to what you were saying, and I made a decision that day to never have sex again until my wedding night."

She then smiled at me and said, "I just want you to know I am now in a committed relationship with a wonderful man, but we are also committed to abstinence. I'm really proud to tell you, I haven't had sex since the day I heard you speak four years ago."

Young people across America who were once involved in sex are waking up to the dangers of this risky behavior and changing their lifestyle. How about you?

If you are disappointed with painful broken relationships, if sex is not what you thought it would be, or if you are worried about the consequences, then maybe it's time to STOP and join the search for *SENSATIONAL SEX*! It's never too late to make *CHOICES* that lead to lifelong success.

Understanding the Difference Between Love and Infatuation

If you are going to make *CHOICES* that lead to lifelong success, you are going to need to understand the difference between love and infatuation. Perhaps the following list will help you think through the differences.

Infatuation usually begins quickly.
Love cultivates slowly and grows steadily throughout the years.

Infatuation tends to focus on one impressive thing about a person.
Love sees the whole person.

Infatuation sees no faults.
Love is aware of the faults and chooses to work through them.

Infatuation does not easily tolerate friends or other activities.
Love encourages friendships and activities.

Infatuation may cause a couple to act more like enemies as they continuously argue.
Love causes a couple to work through conflicts by talking and compromising.

Infatuation causes one to neglect important matters such as school, outside activities, and work.
Love causes one to excel to one's greatest potential.

Infatuation may cause a person to lower his or her standards.
Love uplifts a person and will strengthen one's character.

Infatuation needs to be together at all times.
Love longs to be together but is willing to wait patiently.

Infatuation often focuses on a sexual attraction to each other. Without the physical involvement the relationship would quickly end.
Love may also have strong sexual feelings, but the relationship is based on much more and will continue to grow without physical involvement.

Infatuation often asks the other person to take risks.
Love strives to protect.

Infatuation causes jealousy.
Love brings about trust.

Focus on the Positive

Sexual abstinence is not easy, but it is incredibly freeing. It frees you from:
- Concerns about unwanted pregnancies
- Concerns about STDs
- Concern by the girl about having to "prove her love" to someone she is dating
- Concern by the guy about having sexual advances rejected or feeling pressure to have to make sexual advances at all
- Concern by the girl about her reputation and about the guy bragging to his friends about sex with her
- Feeling like you are just being used for pleasure rather than appreciated for the person you are
- Hiding what's going on in your relationship
- Emotional scars when the relationship ends

Sexual abstinence frees you to:

- Enjoy another person without pressure
- Be yourself in a friendship
- Explore the things you enjoy doing together
- Communicate more honestly with someone as you get to know the real person
- Learn to give to another without selfishly seeking your own pleasure – the basis of any healthy long-term relationship
- Feel good about yourself, your *CHOICES*, and your ability to handle relationships in your life

Read the Fine Print!

> **WARNING:** Sexual abstinence until marriage is not an easy lifestyle. It may be one of the toughest decisions you will ever make in your life. It will require self control, self respect, and self discipline.

The final chapters of this series will provide more suggestions on how to make *CHOICES* that lead to lifelong success. Just be warned:

> Sexual Abstinence
> Is not for Wimps!

Go to **Workbook Chapter 13** beginning on the following page.

How Strong Are You?

1. According to the U.S. Census, the average man gets married at 27 and the average woman gets married at 25. If you made the *CHOICE* to save sex for marriage, how many more years are you going to be waiting? _____

2. Give at least 5 reasons why "Abstinence is not for Wimps!" What struggles and problems make this a challenging lifestyle? Look over Lori's List for additional ideas.

   A._____

   B._____

   C._____

   D._____

   E._____

3. Despite the fact that it is more difficult to save sex for marriage today than ever before, sexual activity among teenagers is dropping for the first time in 25 years. Why do you think most teenagers throughout America are making a decision to postpone sex?

   _____

   _____

   _____

4.   Many adults have laughed at the concept of today's youth saving sex for marriage. They believe it just isn't possible. What do you think? Circle the answer which applies to you.

Sexual abstinence until marriage is going to be:

Impossible   Difficult but possible

5.   If you or one of your friends has already been involved in sex, is it too late to start making *CHOICES* that lead to lifelong success? Explain.

_____

_____

6.   You now have knowledge and understanding about reproduction, fetal development, and sexual intercourse. You know more about STDs than most adults. You are well informed on the leading forms of contraceptives. You've carefully thought through the problems of sex before marriage and the challenges of saving sex for marriage. Now it is time to make *CHOICES*. How are you going to deal with sex? Look again at Lori's List. But this time realize this isn't about Lori any longer. IT'S ABOUT YOU. It's your life, your dreams and your goals. What are you going to do when faced with strong sexual urges? As you look through Lori's List, select the five most important reasons a person would have sex before marriage and put them in the first column of the following chart. Then select the top five compelling reasons a person should save sex for marriage and put them in the second column.

Reasons to Have Sex	Reasons to Save Sex
1.	1.
2.	2.
3.	3.
4.	4.
5.	5.

7. Look carefully at the chart you just completed.

    A.   Which column will more likely provide *Lifelong Success*?

        Reasons to Have Sex   Reasons to Save Sex

    B.   Which column will more likely provide a *Lifetime of Regret*?

        Reasons to Have Sex   Reasons to Save Sex

Family Discussion

1. Discuss the top five reasons you have established as being the "Reasons to Have Sex" and the "Reasons to Save Sex."

2. Sexual abstinence is more difficult today than ever before. So why do you think sexual activity among teenagers is declining?

3. Read the following story and decide if you think Chloe and Conner are experiencing love or infatuation.

        Chloe and Conner met 3 months ago. It was love at first sight. They have been inseparable ever since. Chloe's friends say it must be love since they never see her anymore. Not only did she give up her friends, Chloe also quit drill team. Practice just took too much time away from Conner. Since Chloe gave up her friends, she wished Conner would give up more of his friends. The guys are okay, but she doesn't like the way Conner acts around certain girls. This has sparked a number of fights between them. The fighting isn't fun, but making up is. That's one area which isn't lacking in this relationship. Their love is full of passion. Chloe has determined a little jealousy and fighting are the price one has to pay for love.

Addition Discussion

⇒ If your child has bought into the concept of abstinence until marriage, provide him or her with a Commitment Card. You can make this yourself, design it with your child, or order it from this series. Also consider a Commitment of Love from you to your child. See the sample wording of both certificates in the first section of this book in Chapter 2 under Additional Available Items.

References

[1]Michael, Robert T., et al., *Sex in America*, New York: Little, Brown and Co., 1994; 124.

[2]Ibid., 125.

[3]Associated Press, Washington: "Sex Rate Among Teenage Girls Down for the First Time in 25 Years," *Dallas Morning News*, May 2, 1997. (Note: The article discussed that rates for boys are also down.)

[4]Centers for Disease Control and Prevention, *Morbidity and Mortality Weekly Report*, September 18, 1998; 47:36; 749-752.

[5]Farber, Michael, "Iron Man," *Sports Illustrated*, November, 17, 1997; 87(20):42.

[6]Ryan, Kelly, "Marriage Can Wait, Study Finds," *The Dallas Morning News*; December 5, 1996; 13.

Note to Parents

The last two chapters will provide your children with practical ways to succeed at the abstinent lifestyle. Your children will learn the importance of:

Developing a Dream

Redefining Dating

Setting Boundaries

If your children are going to become successful at developing dreams, they are going to need your constant encouragement and participation. Think back to my story where I talked about my *secret* dream of becoming a professional tennis player. The reason this was my *secret* dream was because I didn't have anyone to dream with.

After the first month of my senior year in high school, I knew my dream of getting married to Chuck was rapidly fading. Not only did I decide to refocus on tennis, I also decided to go on to college and get a degree in education.

For some strange reason I decided to share this dream with my mother. She and I had never spent much time talking together. In fact, this was one of the only heart to heart talks I ever remember having with my mother. I vividly remember sitting at the kitchen table and sharing with her my plan of becoming a teacher. I don't think I had ever seen Mom respond with so much enthusiasm. No doubt the fact that I had chosen to follow in her footsteps as a teacher had something to do with her reaction. For the next hour we talked about the advantages of being a teacher and what I needed to do to accomplish this goal. That was the first and only dream I had ever shared with my mother. Unfortunately, that dream came to an abrupt end a few weeks later when I realized I was pregnant.

> Dream with your children.
> Start early and continue throughout their lives!

Junior high and high school years should be filled with exploring various options for your child's future. One day they might want to be a marine biologist and the next day a doctor or professional athlete. As they develop interest in a certain area, help them see all the possibilities in that field. Have fun as you go to the library or search the Internet together. Talk to various people in the different fields. Remember:

Tool #2

> *CHOICES that Lead to Lifelong Success*
> require
> Learning from Those with Experience

No doubt these dreams will change almost as fast as your child changes clothes, but eventually one will seem to be a perfect fit.

Not only will this chapter encourage your children to learn to become someone special by developing a dream, they will also be encouraged to look at dating in a new and different way. Instead of developing *serious relationships,* they will be challenged to build *sensational friendships* and to set definite boundaries on how far is too far.

You and I both know that *sensational friendships* can quickly turn into *serious relationships*. Well, that is where your child's accountability partner will be of great help. Someone slightly removed from your family can often help your child see when things are getting too serious. There is nothing wrong with letting the accountability partner do a little of your dirty work and save you some grief. Let's face it, teenagers often take constructive criticism better from an outsider than from dear old mom or dad.

A young person who is receiving lots of love from home, who is constantly dreaming with mom and dad about a bright future, and who learns to build sensational friendships with definite boundaries, is a young person who is well on the road to making *CHOICES* that lead to lifelong success!

A Tip from the Tool Box

There is no way to keep your children innocent in today's society. But you can help them become critical thinkers as they learn to look for the good and bad in all situations. For example, when your children go to the movies or read books or magazines, get them in the habit of sharing three positive and three negative points. This will prevent them from mindlessly soaking up information and cause them to continually consider what is going on about them in comparison to your values.

Chapter 14

HOW TO SUCCEED

Knowledge of reproduction and fear of sexually transmitted diseases will not result in sexual abstinence. It's going to take far more than that. If you plan to succeed at making *CHOICES* that lead to lifelong success, you must learn to skillfully use the third and final tool of this series.

Tool #3

Choices that Lead to Lifelong Success
require
Determination to Succeed

In other words, you need to be so committed to sexual abstinence that it becomes a lifestyle. If you are not determined to succeed, you could easily give in to peer pressure and the powerful desire for sex.

Chuck and I said we were committed to abstinence while we were dating, but it was not a passion for either of us. It was merely empty words.

Your passion for abstinence must be able
to withstand the heat of passion

Everybody Needs Somebody

A major problem you are going to face regarding sexual abstinence is the natural desire to have someone special in your life. This often begins in grade school or the early teenage years when everyone seems to be searching for that special person who can fill their needs.

I *need* someone to love me.
I *need* someone to understand me.
I *need* someone to hold and touch
and be a part of my life.
I *need* . . . I *need* . . . I *need*!

As a result, we have become a very *needy* society going from relationship to relationship desperately searching for that special person who will fill our needs. When each relationship ends, there is often pain, resentment, and a greater desire to find someone else to fill our needs.

Perhaps you have seen this situation played out in your school or maybe in your own life. It is like a broken record that won't stop. Everyone keeps dancing to the same music despite the same painful outcome. May I suggest you "stop the music" and consider a different approach.

Instead of trying to find a special person to love and understand you, why don't you learn to love and understand who you are? Instead of spending your time pleasing that special person in hopes of hanging on to them, why not take this time to recognize your own likes and dislikes, your strengths and weaknesses? Set goals and experience the joy of fulfilling your dreams.

How to Stop the Music

If you want to learn how to stop the music and make sure you don't fall into the trap of becoming a needy person, you need to learn how to:

Develop a dream
Redefine dating
Set boundaries

The rest of this book will help you learn how to stop the music and make *CHOICES* that lead to lifelong success.

Develop a Dream

In the final months of high school, most seniors find themselves busy with parties and senior activities. In the midst of all the excitement they are often overwhelmed as they try to answer the following questions:

What am I going to do with the rest of my life?
Am I going to go to college?
What career path do I want to take?

Once in college, many students change their career path more often than they change the sheets on their beds as they desperately try to find a career that feels right.

May I make a suggestion? Why not spend your teenage years determining your strengths and weakness, likes and dislikes? Throughout middle school and high school have fun dreaming with your family and friends as you consider different professions. Consider the following illustration.

When Jack was 11 years old he just knew he wanted to be a fireman. He and his dad visited several fire stations and talked to lots of firemen.

By the time Jack was 14, his dream had changed to baseball. He was showing some real talent on the school team, and his grandfather took him to several professional baseball games.

Although his love for baseball continued, when Jack was 16 he started having thoughts of becoming a lawyer. His aunt worked for an attorney and arranged for him to sit through a trial so he could see what the life of an attorney might be like. After three days in a courtroom, Jack changed his mind and knew that wasn't the direction he wanted to go.

Next, Jack's thoughts turned to medicine. A surgeon attended the same church as Jack's family. So Jack's parents invited him for dinner and Jack spent the evening asking questions.

"What kind of grades are required for medical school? How many years of college will it take? How much money could I make as a doctor? What about the blood; will I ever get used to it? What are the drawbacks of being a doctor?. . ."

The next week the doctor arranged for Jack to watch an operation. Jack knew if he couldn't stomach the blood, he was going to be looking for a new dream. After observing the surgery, Jack had his answer. He wanted to be a doctor more than anything in the world. The thought of saving lives was an awesome feeling.

Jack and his mother immediately began searching the Internet for the best universities which would prepare him for medical school. Soon he knew where he wanted to go and what it was going to take to get there. Jack had always been a decent student, but now he knew "decent" wasn't going to cut it. He had to graduate from high school in the top of his class. He had a little over two years left before graduation to get his grades where they needed to be for entering college. But with his dream in place, now he could focus on fulfilling his goals.

Not only did Jack accomplish his goal of graduating in the top of his class, he also walked away with several awards and helped his baseball team win the district championship.

Jack had a dream and the determination to succeed. How about you? Do you want to be a "needy person" who is desperate to have someone fulfill *your needs* or do you want to be a confident person with dreams and goals and the determination to succeed? The *CHOICE* is yours!

Redefine Dating

If you want to make *CHOICES* that lead to lifelong success, you are going to need to redefine dating. Let's face it. Jack would have found it difficult to get his grades up, graduate in the top of his class, and go on into pre-med if he was distracted with hot and heavy passionate relationships throughout high school.

Does that mean that if you want to succeed you are going to have to avoid dating altogether? No! Go out! Have fun! Go places! Do things! Just avoid passionate relationships. Instead of building serious relationships, spend your time building *sensational friendships*. You can build an incredible relationship with another person by going places together, talking for hours, and laughing together without becoming physically or intimately involved.

Protecting Your Friendships

You need to be careful because a *sensational friendship* can quickly turn into a *serious relationship*. Once this happens, the passion can quickly grow and your vision can become clouded. Then you are suddenly saying crazy things like:

> I *need* you to spend more time with me.
> I *need* you to love me.
> I *need* you to understand me.
> I *need* you to hold me.
> I *need* . . . I *need* . . . I *need*!

Before you know it, you have turned into a needy person and your goal of sexual abstinence can be easily jeopardized as your dreams fade away.

According to a national survey, the second leading reason why teens become involved in sex is a serious relationship.[1] Doesn't that make sense? Two people deeply in love and focused on each other are going to naturally develop passionate feelings for each other. Over a period of time, a simple kiss can turn into heavy passionate kissing . . . soon followed by touching . . . removing clothes . . . and before long, the couple is in the midst of a hot and heavy sexual relationship. If those two people happen to be married, that will make for a very exciting marriage! But if they are not married, they are setting themselves up for problems which can destroy their dreams. Therefore, if you are serious about sexual abstinence, but you aren't ready for marriage then you need to avoid serious relationships.

When you are ready for marriage, a serious relationship will be very exciting. While it may be difficult to control those passionate desires, it will not be impossible if you know your wedding day is near. But if marriage is out of the question, you would be wise to avoid serious relationships so your passion for abstinence is not replaced by the heat of passion.

How do you avoid serious relationships? By setting boundaries.

Setting Boundaries

If you are going to succeed at saving sex for marriage and fulfilling exciting dreams, you are going to need to **set definite boundaries to determine how far is too far**. As you consider this, you need to realize that sex is far more than sexual intercourse. No doubt you have seen this on television and in the movies. A sexual encounter usually begins with hot passionate kissing and then progresses as follows:

Passionate Kissing

Intimate Touching

Removing Clothes

Sexual Intercourse

Each of these steps prepares the couple both physically and mentally for sexual intercourse.

A young lady once told me she and her boyfriend had been dating for three years and were committed to abstinence. Then one night they suddenly had sex. This sounded strange, so I questioned her further. "You mean the two of you had been completely committed to abstinence for three years, and then one night, without warning, you had sex?"

"Yes," she replied.

This still sounded strange so I questioned her further. "You mean you had never kissed passionately, touched under clothes, or removed your clothes?"

"Oh sure, we had done all that. But we were committed to abstinence."

No. They were not committed to abstinence. Everything they were doing was preparing their minds and bodies for sexual intercourse. By kissing passionately, touching intimately, removing clothes and then suddenly stopping, this couple was no doubt feeling tremendous frustration. This frustration was going to eventually cause them to break up or go all the way. (I should know; that is exactly what happened to me.)

The Solution

Those who are serious about a lifestyle of sexual abstinence before marriage should avoid the natural progression of sexual intercourse altogether. That means avoiding the very first step of heavy, passionate kissing. Although you may have no intentions of going any further, you will soon find yourself caught up in the natural progression, desiring the next step. Then you will begin telling yourself things like, "Kissing never hurt anything." That will soon be followed by, "A little touching won't hurt us."

Warning: Don't underestimate the powerful sex drive!

> If you do not control your sex drive,
> it will control you!

What About a Kiss?

Is one kiss okay? What about two or three kisses? A dozen? The real question you need to answer is this: Can you remain in control of your thoughts and your heart with a kiss or two? Even if you think you could (and almost no one can), the next question to ask is this: Will kissing suddenly take this *sensational friendship* to the next stage, a *serious relationship*? If the answer to this question is yes, you need to determine if you are ready for a serious relationship. Remember, if you aren't ready for marriage, you aren't ready for a serious relationship.

Perhaps at this point it would be wise to remind you that I never said abstinence is an easy lifestyle. Remember:

> Sexual Abstinence is not for Wimps!

Building a Foundation

When a building is being constructed, the foundation is critical. Without a solid foundation the walls and roof can easily collapse.

Marriages are also built on foundations. If the foundation is not strong and solid, the marriage can collapse under the pressures and stress of life.

Today, many marriages begin with a foundation of *passion*. Two people meet and immediately experience a physical attraction. Their passion is quickly unleashed. This might be through hot and heavy kissing or actually having sex. Either way, the foundation of passion has been established. A passionate relationship usually moves quickly into a *serious relationship* and in time may end up in *marriage*.

The problem is that passion alone produces a weak foundation. After only a few years of marriage, the couple realizes they have nothing in common. Little things begin to annoy them as they ask, "Who is this person I'm married to?" Soon, the very foundation of passion which once held them together begins to fade. When problems come, as they always do in life, the cracked and crumbled foundation of passion has trouble holding the couple together under the stress and strain of life. Divorce often follows.

The progression of a relationship based on *PASSION* often resembles the following pattern:

➡ P A S S I O N
　　➡ Serious Relationship
　　　➡ Marriage
　　　　➡ Who is this person I'm married to?

Marriages which begin with the foundation of *friendship* are different. When a couple controls their sexual desires and develops a sensational friendship as the foundation, they actually end up marrying their best friend. They know each other intimately before marriage, but NOT physically. *After* marriage they unleash their passion as they become lovers *inside* marriage. When problems come, as they always do in life, the foundation of best friends may be tested by the stress and strains of life, but the marriage is far more likely to stand firm because of the strong foundation of *friendship*.

The progression of a relationship based on *FRIENDSHIP* often resembles the following pattern:

➡ B E S T   F R I E N D S
 ➡ Serious Relationship
  ➡ Marriage
   ➡ Passion

Which foundation would you prefer your marriage to be built upon? A foundation of passion or a foundation of best friends? The *CHOICES* you make can lead to lifelong success or a lifetime of regret.

Go to **Workbook Chapter 14** beginning on the following page.

Stop the Music

1. Tool #3 states:

   "CHOICES that Lead to Lifelong Success require

   _____ "

2. Have you heard yourself say the following?
   I *need* a boyfriend/girlfriend.
   I *need* someone to love me.
   I *need* to hold someone.

   After reading this chapter, would you say you have experienced the situation of being a needy person? Explain.

   _____

   _____

   _____

3. In this chapter you learned that if you want to protect yourself from becoming a *needy* person you must:

   Develop a _____

   Redefine _____

   Set _____

4. If you had to decide right now what you were going to do for the rest of your life, what would it be?

   My dream in life is to be a _____

5. If you want to make sure you are successful at fulfilling your dreams, you are going to need to redefine dating. Write three guidelines to dating which will help you make *CHOICES* that lead to lifelong success. It might help to start your sentences

with the words "I will" or "I will not."

A._____

B._____

C._____

6. If you want to make sure you fulfill your dreams, you are also going to need to set definite boundaries by deciding how far is too far. Draw a line at the point where you plan to stop from this day forward to protect yourself from pregnancies, STDs, and emotional scars. (It does not matter what you have done in the past. This is about the boundaries you plan to set starting today.)

Talk

Hold Hands

Hug and Kiss

Passionate Kissing

Touch Under Clothes

Remove Your Clothing

Have Sexual Intercourse

7. As you build sensational friendships you need to be on your guard for risky situations which could quickly move that friendship into a serious relationship. Put an "R" by the following date ideas that are risky and an "S" by the safer ideas.

_____ Playing tennis
_____ Riding bikes
_____ Baby sitting together
_____ Rock climbing
_____ Jogging

_____	Watching TV at home all alone
_____	Eating at the food court at the mall
_____	Going to a party where alcohol is served
_____	Meeting a group of friends for coffee
_____	Going to a baseball game
_____	Swimming together all alone

Family Discussion

1. If you want to make sure you do not become a needy person, you will need to develop a dream. Remember, that dream can change as often as necessary until you find the dream that really fits. Share with your parents the dream you selected in your workbook and write it in the blank below. Then, as a family, discuss and write down 10 things you need to do to succeed with that dream.

   How to succeed with my dream of becoming a _____

   1)_____

   2)_____

   3)_____

   4)_____

   5)_____

   6)_____

   7)_____

   8)_____

   9)_____

   10)_____

Don't forget to add Tool #2 to your list:

Tool #2

> *Choices that Lead to Lifelong Success*
> require
> Learning from Those with Experience

2. Write down three things you can begin doing this week to make this dream come true. (These are your short-term goals.)

    1)_____

    2)_____

    3)_____

3. Now write down at least three things you would like to accomplish in the next year to help fulfill your dreams. (These become your one-year goals.)

    1)_____

    2)_____

    3)_____

4. Now write down at least three things you will need to accomplish within the next 5 years to make this dream come true. (These are your long-term goals.)

    1)_____

    2)_____

    3)_____

Congratulations! You are now well on your way to achieving this dream! If the dream changes, go through this same process again to establish the necessary goals. Reminders on your mirror or refrigerator might help you check the progress of your goals on a regular basis. Don't forget:

Tool #3

CHOICES that Lead to Lifelong Success
require
Determination to Succeed

Additional Discussion

⇒ If a couple is committed to sexual abstinence until marriage, could passionate kissing be dangerous? Explain.

⇒ Explain where you decided to draw the line to make sure you don't face a pregnancy, STDs, or emotional scars.

⇒ Discuss at least 10 fun things a couple can do that would not be risky.

⇒ Discuss the differences between building a relationship on the foundation of Best Friends and the foundation of Passion.

⇒ Why is sexual abstinence NOT for wimps?

References

[1]Small, Stephen A., and Luster, Tom, "Adolescent Sexual Activity," *Journal of Marriage and the Family*, February 1994; 181-192.

Note to Parents

Congratulations, you made it to the final chapter!

This chapter is filled with creative suggestions to help your children successfully live the abstinent lifestyle. But don't think that just because you have concluded this series your work is over. It is important that you continue to challenge and encourage your children. Even as they leave home and go off to college or start a career, they are going to need your encouragement and support. Students have told me sexual pressures are far greater after high school than during it.

A lady told me her father first started encouraging her with the concept of sexual abstinence when she was 12 years old. She said she remembered the night he came in her room to tell her good night and said, "Honey, I want to tell you about the most wonderful gift your mother ever gave me. This was a gift she gave me the night we got married. It was the gift of her virginity." As he reached down to kiss her cheek, he said, "I hope you value yourself and your virginity enough to save yourself for your husband."

About a year later she said she and her dad were in the car driving down the road when he said, "Honey, I want to tell you about the most precious gift your mother ever gave me . . ." Once again he told the story.

As the years went by she heard that story over and over. Years later she realized her father must have selected the month of her birthday to serve as a reminder to have their little talk, because year after year she heard the same story. Even after she went off to college the talk continued. She said she would be in her dorm room, the phone would ring, and on the other end of the line she would hear her father saying, "Honcy, I wanted to tell you about the most precious gift your mother ever gave me . . . "

The lady said after graduating from college she married a wonderful man, and yes, her father's persistence paid off. On her wedding night she gave her husband the gift of her virginity. She went on to say that recently she was about to tell her daughter good night when she overheard her husband's voice coming from their daughter's bedroom. He was saying, "Honey, I want to tell you about the most precious gift your mother ever gave me. It was a gift she gave me on our wedding night . . ."

To be successful, the message of sexual abstinence until marriage must continue through the years. Be creative and find a way to start a tradition with your children, one that could be passed down from generation to generation.

I encourage you to go through this series again in another year or two. You can have fun comparing the answers with those from previous years. Although the information in the series will not change, your family discussion will probably grow deeper each time you go through it.

The organization I am with, Aim for Success, Inc., provides a one-page mailing for parents called *Tips on Encouraging Sexual Purity*. Each month new information is provided regarding the latest statistics on STDs, personal stories, or other pertinent information which can help you continue to encourage your children toward sexual abstinence. If you would like more information about receiving this monthly mailing, call Aim for Success at (972) 422-2322.

A Tip from the Tool Box

According to a national study conducted by the U.S. government, teens who place importance on religion and prayer are less likely than others to smoke, drink alcohol, and use marijuana. They are also more likely to delay sexual activity.[1] If your family has religious values, this can have a significant impact on your child's success in this lifestyle. Encourage your child to memorize scripture which deals with this subject, and pray for your child's strength and protection. Pray also for your child's future spouse and the *CHOICES* he or she will be making about sexual activity.

[1]Resnick, Michael. D, Ph.D., et al., "Protecting Adolescents from Harm: Findings from the National Longitudinal Study on Adolescent Health," *Journal of the American Medical Association,* 9/10/97.

Chapter 15

DEVELOPING HIGH STANDARDS

A young lady who had just graduated from high school told me, "Every time I tell a boy no, my virginity becomes a little more valuable and my self-image moves up another notch." High standards and good self-image go hand-in-hand.

But developing the high standard of sexual abstinence is not easy, especially in this sex-saturated society. A high school senior and member of the football team phrased it very well when he told me, "It's really tough staying committed to abstinence today, especially when girls seem to want it more than the guys."

Developing high standards can also bring ridicule. A.C. Green is a perfect example of this. As previously discussed, A.C. Green holds the NBA record for the most consecutive games played. Even in college it was well known that he was a virgin and was committed to sexual abstinence until marriage. In an effort to distract his concentration, rival fans would hold up centerfolds of nude women while he shot free throws. No wonder *Sports Illustrated* called him the "Iron Man."[1]

How to Develop High Standards

Be careful about alcohol and drugs. Alcohol is the number one reason why teenagers have sex.[2] Think about it. Alcohol and drugs cause a person to lose self control. Self control is the most important ingredient in succeeding at the abstinent lifestyle.

Abstinence and alcohol do not mix!
One requires self-control, the other destroys it.

293

Be careful to state your stand early in a relationship. Be honest, open and proud of your stand on sexual abstinence. Let your friends and each person you date know about your commitment from the very beginning.

Be careful to have definite boundaries. Know exactly what you will and will not do. When it comes to physical involvement, consider the "The 3 Nothings Rule."

The 3 Nothings Rule

Nothing below the neck.
Nothing under clothes.
Nothing lying down.

Be careful to date like-minded people. If the person you are dating is not committed to sexual abstinence, there is a good chance that person will cause you to question your stand. You could soon find yourself compromising your commitment. That person is much more likely to bring you down than you are to bring them up to your standards.

Be careful how you dress. Girls, this is especially important for you. Boys are turned on by sight; girls are turned on by touch. It takes very little to make a boy think you want to have sex. When a girl walks in a room with short shorts and a tight top on, she can drive guys crazy. This is not necessarily a compliment. The fact is *any girl* can turn *any guy* on. If you wear seductive clothing you are either teasing your boyfriend, which is very cruel, or giving him an open invitation to get physical. Neither of these are going to help you succeed at sexual abstinence.

It may take some effort, but you can dress stylishly without being seductive. This includes anything from formals to bathing suits. When I recently bought a new skirt, I tried it on for my husband and asked him if he thought it was too short. He said that although it was shorter than my other skirts, he thought it was still tasteful.

I recommend you ask your father, uncle, or brother to give you their opinion on the clothes you buy. What you and your girlfriends might really like, guys might see as seductive.

> By wearing seductive clothes,
> you are either teasing your boyfriend
> or giving him an open invitation.

Be careful how you touch. This is especially true for boys. Men, you need to remember girls are turned on by touch. A 19-year-old girl told me she almost lost it when her boyfriend gave her a foot massage. Who would ever think of touching someone's feet as a turn on, but on that particular evening it certainly was for her. Remember, once you turn on, it can be very difficult to turn off.

Be careful when you're feeling vulnerable. If you are feeling weak or vulnerable, get out of the situation. For example, if holding hands one evening is really turning you on, tell the person you can't do that right now. Remember, there are a few days each month when girls are more easily aroused. Boys, on the other hand, are ready for sexual arousal 365 days a year. If you learn to be considerate of each other, it will keep your frustration level at a minimum.

Be careful to respect the word "NO!" The word "no" never means maybe or yes. It always means no. If the person you are with says "no," then stop.

Be careful where you go. Find a safe place to be together. This should not be your bedroom. I'm amazed at how many teenagers spend hours together in bedrooms playing computer games and watching television. Remember, the sex drive is very powerful, and the bedroom is not safe! Try the family room, or if you want to be alone, go to the food court at the mall or take a walk in the park. There are safe ways of being alone without being completely alone.

Be careful what you watch. Television and the movies are often filled with explicit sexual scenes. Watching gorgeous Hollywood actors having hot and heavy sex is not going to help your self control.

Be careful of pornography. Looking at magazines and videos of beautiful naked bodies will *destroy* your ability to control your sexual desires. Remember, as you admire these gorgeous bodies you are feeding your sexual appetite and losing your self control. **Warning:** pornography can become an addiction! A man told me his college roommate introduced him to pornography. At the time it was fun and exciting. Today, it is an addiction which has cost him his job and his family. He has lost virtually everything that was important to him. His case is not uncommon. This has become such a serious problem that support groups for it are spreading throughout the country.

> Pornography feeds your sexual appetite
> and destroys self-control.

Be careful of what you see and do on the Internet. The Internet, even chat rooms, can be just as pornographic as any X-rated video. If you are serious about controlling your sexual appetite, you need to guard what you feed your mind.

Be careful about satisfying your sexual desires by masturbating. Is masturbating bad? No. There is nothing wrong with wanting to understand how your body works. But to release sexual tension by masturbating requires concentrating on sexual fantasies. Remember, the goal of sexual abstinence is self control. This includes keeping thoughts and actions under control. Therefore, a person who masturbates on a regular basis is not gaining control over his or her thought life, but is feeding it with sensual thoughts. More than likely this will not satisfy for long, and soon the person will be desiring more than masturbation.

Two Common Questions

What if I save myself for marriage, but the person I want to marry is not a virgin? This could happen. The person you fall in love with may have been sexually active then somewhere along the way made a commitment to abstinence. After all, many previously sexually active teenagers are now changing their lifestyle and making a commitment to abstinence. If you find yourself in this situation, try the "Three-Way Test."

1. Ask the person to be tested for STDs. If there are problems, you will need to determine how it will affect you and whether you can live with the problem.

2. Look for emotional scars. Determine if you can live with the problems which have resulted from their past. Then consider how you will feel knowing you are not his or her first and only partner.

3. Finally, and most importantly, determine if the person has really changed. Is there now a genuine commitment to abstinence? Do you see a pattern of self control and self discipline, or could this be a temporary change just to please you and win you over? If it is real, you will see a determination to succeed at abstinence and strong evidence of self control in other areas of their life.

What if I never get married? First of all, this would be rare. In fact, 90% of all Americans get married by age 30.[3] If, however, you are serious about sexual abstinence until marriage, there is a slight chance you might never marry and never experience sex. But in exchange, you will be guaranteed freedom from STDs, unplanned pregnancies, and painful emotional scars. You will also gain a tremendous amount of strength and self control and build many strong friendships. I personally know single people of all ages committed to abstinence who are living extremely successful lives without sex.

Additional Helpful Suggestions

Put your commitment in writing. Teenagers who take a pledge to remain a virgin until marriage are more likely to delay intercourse.[4] Write out your own commitment and consider having it matted and framed; or order a certificate from this series. Information about commitment certificates is provided in the Parent Introduction.

Find an accountability partner. This should be someone several years older than you, someone who believes in you and cares deeply for your well-being. This should also be a person who can sense when you are headed in the wrong direction and someone you highly respect.

Stay focused on your dreams and goals. Whether your dream is to become a football player, dancer, model, veterinarian, attorney, teacher, doctor, or marine biologist you need to stay focused on your goals.

Make a habit of developing short-term and long-term goals. Share your goals with your parents and accountability partner and have fun dreaming together about your future.

> If you are focused on your dreams
> everyone will know where you are headed.

Find like-minded friends. Sexual abstinence is much easier when you hang around a group of friends who have the same commitment.

Give of yourself. Studies have shown that teenagers who are committed to community service projects are less likely to be sexually active. Volunteer your time at the hospital, the homeless shelter, or a nursing home. Do yard work or clean house for an elderly person.

Wear a commitment ring, necklace, or bracelet. This can serve as a reminder to you and to those you date of your commitment to sexual abstinence. Taking this a step further, you can replace the commitment rings during the wedding ceremony with your wedding rings. After you are pronounced 'Husband and Wife' and you turn to walk down the aisle, the groom can hand the bride's commitment ring to her parents and she can return the groom's ring to his parents. In years to come, these commitment rings could be passed on to your children.

Write a love letter to your future spouse. In a love letter to your future spouse explain in detail why you have decided to save yourself for your wedding night. Date and sign the letter then save it for your wedding night. What a great gift! (When you find yourself feeling weak, take the letter out and read it as a way to strengthen your commitment.)

Buy your future spouse gifts. Show your future spouse how much you thought of him or her long before you ever met each other. Start buying your spouse one special gift a year. (It doesn't need to be expensive, just meaningful. Perhaps a CD with a special song, a postcard or poster of a romantic scene, etc.) Wrap each gift with the date and a note explaining why this particular gift made you think of him or her. Then during your first year of marriage present your spouse with one of the gifts on your one month anniversary. Then give another gift on your second month anniversary, etc.

Make a list of "I will not..." For example, I will not date anyone who is not committed to sexual abstinence. I will not drink alcohol or do drugs. Be very specific with your list. Share your list with your parents and your accountability partner. Once a year, perhaps on your birthday, review the list together.

Know what your religion says about sex before marriage. Most religions have strong convictions about sexual abstinence until marriage. Spiritual faith can be a major element in succeeding at this lifestyle. Pray for strength and protection. Study and memorize scripture which deals with sexual abstinence.

When you feel weak, review Lori's List from your workbook. Remind yourself of all the reasons you don't want to get physically involved.

If you stumble, don't stay down! Get right back up and continue on. A 28-year-old woman told me that she made a commitment to sexual abstinence when she was 13. She was pleased when she graduated from high school as a virgin, but when she graduated from college as a virgin she was downright proud!

When she was 26 years old she met a very nice 30-year-old man. On the first date she explained to him her commitment to sexual abstinence – just as she had done with all the other men before him. He told her he respected her stand. But a few weeks later he took her in his arms, kissed her, and told her it was time to put away her childish ideas and become a woman. In a moment of passion and weakness, she gave up her virginity.

Immediately, she knew it was a terrible mistake and regretted what she had done. Fortunately, there was no pregnancy and no diseases. In her determination to protect herself from ongoing emotional scars, she forgave herself and recommitted herself to sexual abstinence until marriage. It's been two years since that evening, and while she deeply regrets her moment of weakness, she is more committed than ever to sexual abstinence until marriage.

Regard your virginity as a priceless gift, not an embarrassing label. *Be proud of being a virgin* and don't be ashamed to let others know where you stand. Being a virgin does not make you an outcast. Most junior high and high school students today are virgins. Your courage to take a strong stand for abstinence may literally save your life and other lives as well. If you aren't a virgin, you can still be proud of your commitment to abstinence and be a positive role model to others!

Reaping the Rewards

As you strive for *SENSATIONAL SEX* you need to remember sexual abstinence is going to be a very difficult lifestyle. You will need to buy into the concept 100 percent if you want to ensure success. The rewards you will gain by living this lifestyle will influence all areas of your life and the benefits will last a lifetime. A few of the rewards you can expect are:

Self Control.
A disciplined life.
A positive example.
Fulfilled dreams and goals.
No pregnancy before marriage.
Respect for yourself and for others.
No guilt of infecting others with an STD.
No STDs producing painful, recurring sores.
No painful memories of past sexual encounters.
Ability to tell your children you waited until marriage.

Becoming a GREAT LOVER!

I once heard an eighty-year-old man being interviewed on the radio. He was asked, "Sir, when does a man stop enjoying sex?" The old man responded in a feeble voice, "I don't know, but when I get there I will let you know."

Look forward to your wedding night with great anticipation. But remember, becoming a great lover takes time. Consider making love as a form of art. Art takes time, patience, and practice to perfect. So be patient as the two of you work together and learn the art of making love. What you will find is that sex will get better and better as the years go by. This is one area where practice really does make perfect.

So give yourself time to perfect the art of making love. After all, what's the hurry? The two of you have a lifetime to develop *SENSATIONAL SEX* while you *practice, practice, practice*!

Go to the next page and complete **Workbook Chapter 15**.

Raising the Standard

1. Write the most compelling reasons that caused you to make a commitment to sexual abstinence or kept you from making this commitment.

    _____

    _____

    _____

    _____

2. Look through the list of "Be Careful" suggestions from this chapter. List five that will be most helpful as you make your *CHOICES*.

    A._____

    B._____

    C._____

    D._____

    E._____

3. If you are making a commitment to abstinence, circle the following ways you plan to help yourself succeed.

    A. Sign a Commitment Certificate.

    B. Find an accountability partner.

    C. Stay focused on your dreams and goals.

    D. Find like-minded friends.

    E. Give of yourself through service projects.

F.　　Wear a commitment ring, necklace or bracelet.

G.　　Write a love letter to your future spouse.

H.　　Buy your future spouse gifts.

I.　　Make a list of "I will not . . ."

J.　　Study what your religion says about sex before marriage.

K.　　Look over Lori's List when feeling weak.

L.　　Don't stay down if you stumble.

M.　　Regard your virginity as a priceless gift, not an embarrassing label.

4.　　Are there any other ideas which would help you succeed at the abstinent lifestyle?

_____

_____

_____

5.　　On a piece of paper, write down each idea you circled. Put that list on your mirror or in a drawer as a reminder of what you need to be doing to succeed at abstinence.

6.　　Complete the following:
I finished this series on (date) _____

Now that I have finished, I feel this series was:

_____

_____

_____

7.   If you have made a commitment to sexual abstinence, let your parents or the person who gave this series to you know about your decision during the Family Discussion.

Closing Notes

Congratulations! You made it to the end of this series. Whether you made a commitment to abstinence or not, hopefully you have learned a great deal about making *CHOICES*.
Remember,

CHOICES that Lead to Lifelong Success require:

Tool # 1 – Knowledge and Understanding
Tool # 2 – Learning from Those with Experience
Tool # 3 – Determination to Succeed

You now have the knowledge and understanding to make wise *CHOICES* about sex. You can apply these same tools to any decision you make in life. The *CHOICES* you make can lead to lifelong success or a lifetime of regret. The *CHOICE* is yours!

Family Discussion

1.   In this chapter you were encouraged to develop high standards. You were also given a list of areas to "Be careful of." Go through that list and discuss what you think are the two or three areas guys need to be most careful about and the two or three which girls need to be most careful about.

2.   If your family has religious values, discuss what your religion says regarding sex before marriage. In what ways could you and your parents be praying for you and your future spouse?

3.   You need to be prepared for sexual advances by others. What would you say if someone said to you:

  • "Come on. Everyone's having sex!"
  • "If you love me you'd have sex with me."
  • "If you were a real man you'd have sex with me."
  • "It's okay, I have protection."

(Some suggested ideas are in the back of this book.)

4.   What would you do if:

  • You were invited to a party and several people were drinking and doing drugs? Explain.

  • You were with some friends and they started looking through magazines with nude bodies or wanted to watch a video with explicit sex scenes?

  • One night you went past the boundaries you had set?

  • You were feeling very weak and not sure you could continue the abstinent lifestyle any longer?

Congratulations! You have now finished this book. In closing, discuss your overall opinion:

  • Has this book expanded your knowledge and understanding of sex?

  • Can you talk together about sex more comfortably now than when you first started?

  • In five years from now, what do you think you will remember most about what you have learned?

  • Has this book helped you make *CHOICES* that lead to lifelong success? Explain.

- Now that you have completed this book, take a minute and see how much you have learned. On the next page is a copy of the pretest you took when you first started. As a family, take the test again and see how much knowledge and understanding you have gained.

If this book has been beneficial to you and your family, I would love to hear from you. Drop me a note at:

Aim for Success, Inc.
P.O. Box 550336
Dallas, TX 75355-0336
or
CHOICES@aim-for-success.org

Test Your Knowledge

This is the same test you took in the beginning of this series. Try taking the test again and see how much you have learned. The answers are in the back of this book under "Chapter 1 – Pretest."

Answer the following questions:

1. Can a girl become pregnant without sexual intercourse?
    A. It is impossible.
    B. It is possible but not likely.
    C. It is very possible.

2. A person can get a sexually transmitted disease without having sexual intercourse.
    A. It is impossible.
    B. It is possible but not likely.
    C. It is very possible.

3. Once a guy reaches the teenage years he produces how many sperm?
    A. About one hundred million sperm a day
    B. About one hundred million sperm a year
    C. About one hundred million sperm in a lifetime

4. A female has the most eggs for reproduction when she is
    A. Inside her mother's womb
    B. 15 years old
    C. 25 years old

5. Approximately how many sexually active teenagers get a sexually transmitted disease each year?
    A. 1 out of 2 sexually active teenagers
    B. 1 out of 4 sexually active teenagers
    C. 1 out of 10 sexually active teenagers
    D. 1 out of 20 sexually active teenagers

6. Most people with sexually transmitted diseases
    A. Have painful sores
    B. Have painless sores
    C. Have sores, a rash, fever and/or pain while urinating
    D. Have no sores or any symptoms at all

7. Which of the following sexually transmitted diseases can lead to death? (There may be more than one.)
    A. AIDS
    B. Gonorrhea
    C. Human Papilloma Virus
    D. Hepatitis B

Additional Discussion

⇒ Whether your children made a commitment to sexual abstinence or not, let them know how proud you are of them for completing this series.

⇒ If your children made a commitment to abstinence, let them know you will be by their side, providing encouragement and support. Remind your children that your love does not depend on the success of this commitment

References

[1]Farber, Michael, "Iron Man," *Sports Illustrated*, November, 17, 1997; 87(20):42.

[2]Small, Stephen A., and Luster, Tom, "Adolescent Sexual Activity," *Journal of Marriage and the Family*, February 1994; 181-192.

[3]Michael, Robert T., et al., *Sex in America*, New York: Little, Brown and Co., 1994.

[4]Resnick, M.D. et al., Protecting Adolescents from Harm – Findings from the National Longitudinal Study on Adolescent Health. *Journal of the American Medical Association*, September 1997; 278 (10), 823-832.

GLOSSARY

GLOSSARY

GLOSSARY

Abortion –Premature extraction of an embryo or fetus from the uterus.

Abstain – To voluntarily do without or refrain from something desired. (For example, a person may choose to abstain from smoking, drinking, drugs, and sex.)

Abstinence – The act of voluntarily doing without certain pleasures.

Abuse – To intentionally hurt or offend another person. There are various forms of abuse: verbal, physical, or sexual.

Abuser – A person who abuses another person. This could be a stranger, acquaintance or family member.

Acquired Immune Deficiency Syndrome (AIDS) – A disease caused by the Human Immunodeficiency Virus (HIV). It destroys the immune system, leaving the infected person unable to fight off certain opportunistic infections.

Adolescence – The stage in life between childhood and adulthood.

Adoption – To bring a child who was born to someone else into a home and raise as a family member.

Anal – Of or relating to the anus.

Anus – The outer rectal opening between the buttocks. This opening remains closed except during defecation (when a person has a bowel movement).

Asymptomatic – No signs, no symptoms but contagious. Most people with sexually transmitted diseases are asymptomatic.

Birth Canal – The passage a baby travels during the birth process. Also known as the vagina.

Birth Control – The use of certain devices to control the number of children a person has.

Birth Control Pill – A pill taken by women to prevent pregnancy.

Bisexual – Attracted sexually to both men and women.

Breast – Female mammary gland used to produce milk for newborn babies.

Cervical Cancer – A malignant tumor in the cervix. It can be caused by a sexually transmitted disease, human papilloma virus (HPV).

Cervix – The opening of the uterus.

313

Cesarean Section – A surgical procedure to deliver a baby when a normal vaginal delivery is not possible. This requires an incision through the abdominal wall and uterus.

Chancre – A painless sore. Syphilis begins with a chancre at the sight where the bacteria infected the body. This is usually the genital area, mouth, or lips. Although the sore will disappear, the person will still be infected until treated with proper medication.

Chlamydia – A bacterial sexually transmitted disease which can cause infertility. Known as the silent sterilizer.

Chromosomes – Strands within a cell's nucleus that contain genetic information. In human reproduction the male and female each provide 23 chromosomes. These 46 chromosomes determine the child's sex, height, color of eyes and hair as well as other features.

Climax – An orgasm or peak of sexual excitement. Accompanied by ejaculation for the male.

Clitoris – A small, sensitive organ which gives sexual stimulation to a female. It is located above the vaginal opening.

Coitus – Sexual intercourse.

Conception – The penetration of the sperm into the egg (ovum). This usually occurs in the fallopian tube. Also called fertilization.

Condom – A thin balloon-like latex covering which fits snugly over a man's penis during sexual intercourse. It is used to help reduce (but not eliminate) the chance of sexually transmitted diseases and pregnancy.

Consequence – The logical result of an action.

Contraceptive – A device or method used to prevent a pregnancy.

Crabs – A slang term for pubic lice. These annoying tiny creatures cause intense itching and irritation of the skin, usually around the pubic (genital) area. They are usually spread by sexual intercourse, sexual contact or the bed sheets of an infected person.

Date Rape – Forced sexual intercourse by an acquaintance.

Depo-Provera – An injection which prevents pregnancy for three months.

Dry Sex – Physical activity which stops just before sexual intercourse. Used by some to prevent pregnancy. However, if sperm is near the vaginal opening a pregnancy could still occur. A person could also become infected with an STD while engaging in dry sex.

Dysplasia – Pre-cancerous cells.

Ectopic Pregnancy – A fertilized egg implanting somewhere other than the uterus, usually in the fallopian tube. Also known as a tubal pregnancy.

Egg – Reproductive cell produced by the female. Also called ovum. Contains the mother's hereditary material in 23 chromosomes.

Ejaculation – The process by which sperm leaves the male body. This can result from sexual excitement or nocturnal emission.

Embryo – The term used for an unborn baby during the earliest stages of development, usually conception until the eighth week.

Epididymis – A thin tightly coiled tube about 20 feet long in the testicles used to store sperm.

Erection – The state of a man's penis becoming rigid or stiff. This is the result of blood filling the inside of the penis. Normally, a man's penis is soft, but it must be erect during sexual intercourse so it can be inserted into the woman's vagina.

Estrogen – A female sex hormone which causes breast development and menstruation.

Fallopian Tubes – Two slender, delicate tubes which transport the egg from the ovary to the uterus. This is where conception usually takes place.

Female – A girl or a woman. The opposite of a male.

Fertile – Capable of reproducing. Men are always fertile and women are fertile only one or two days each month. Women will stop being fertile around age 50 while men continue to be fertile.

Fertilization – The penetration of the sperm into the egg (ovum). This usually occurs in the fallopian tube. Also called conception.

Fetus – The term used to refer to an unborn baby from the eighth week of pregnancy until birth. This is a Latin term for "young one" or "offspring."

Fraternal Twins – Twins which result from two eggs being released and fertilized by two sperm. They could be the same sex or a boy and a girl.

Genitals – Sexual organs or the sexual area of a male or female.

Genital Herpes – A common sexually transmitted disease usually caused by herpes simplex virus type 2 (HSV2). This incurable disease can cause painful reoccurring blisters and sores in the genital area.

Gestation – The length of a pregnancy.

Gonads – The sex glands which send out hormones that cause growth and changes in the body. These are the ovaries in females and testicles in males.

Gonorrhea – A pus-producing bacterium which is transmitted by sexual contact.

Hepatitis B – A common viral sexually transmitted disease which can cause liver cancer. There is no cure for this virus, but there is a vaccine to prevent the infection.

Herpes – An incurable sexually transmitted disease which causes painful blisters and sores. Herpes Simplex Type 1 generally produces sores around the mouth while Herpes Simplex Type 2 usually produces sores in the genital area.

Heterosexual – A person who is sexually attracted to those of the opposite sex.

HIV (Human Immunodeficiency Virus) – The virus which causes Acquired Immune Deficiency Syndrome (AIDS).

Homosexual – A person who is sexually attracted to those of the same sex.

Human Papilloma Virus (HPV) – A highly contagious, incurable sexually transmitted disease which may result in genital warts and cancer.

Hysterectomy – Surgical removal of the uterus.

Identical Twins – Twins which are produced when the fertilized egg splits for unknown reasons. Both eggs have identical genes. These children will always be the same sex and look alike.

Infertile – Not able to reproduce.

Labia Majora – Two outer folds of skin which cover the female genital area.

Labia Minora – Two small folds of mucus membrane inside the larger folds of the labia majora.

Male – A boy or a man. The opposite of a female.

Masturbation – To manipulate one's own sexual organs to bring sexual pleasure.

Menarche – The first menstrual period of a girl in puberty. Usually around 10 to 14 years of age.

Menopause – When menstruation ceases for a woman, usually around age 50.

Menstruation – The process by which the lining of the uterus is discarded as a bloody discharge. This occurs about every 28 days for women and lasts for 3 to 7 days. A woman will menstruate about 400 times during her life.

Miscarriage – The unintentional termination of a pregnancy before the twentieth week.

Monogamous – The practice of having only one mate.

Mutual Masturbation – To manipulate another person's sexual organs to bring sexual pleasure. Considered by some as a safe way to enjoy sexual pleasure. However, this can spread STDs if one of the partners is infected.

Nocturnal Emission – The body's natural way of releasing the build-up of sperm. This happens while a male sleeps and is very normal. Also called "wet dream."

Norplant - Six matchstick-size implants inserted under the skin of a woman's upper arm to prevent pregnancy. Protection lasts for five years.

Oral Sex – Sexual gratification of the genitals by using the lips and mouth.

Orgasm – The state of physical and emotional excitement that occurs at the climax of sexual intercourse. In the male it is accompanied by ejaculation of semen.

Ovaries – The female reproductive organs where the eggs are stored. There is one ovary on each side of the uterus inside the lower abdomen of a woman. The ovaries also produce the female sex hormones, estrogen and progesterone.

Ovulation – The process of the ovary releasing an egg or ovum.

Ovum – The egg released by the female which contains the mother's hereditary material in 23 chromosomes.

Pap Smear – A test in which a smear of secretions from the cervix and vagina are taken to test for abnormal cells. This test can detect early stages of cancer in women.

Pelvic Inflammatory Disease (PID) – An infection of the uterus, fallopian tubes or ovaries. It is the most common complication of sexually transmitted diseases. It can result in chronic pain, sterility, and ectopic pregnancies.

Penetrate – To go inward; to pierce, as when a man's penis penetrates the woman's vagina, or a sperm penetrates the egg at conception.

Penis – The male sex organ. It is located on the outside of the body and is used to transport urine and semen from the body.

Period – Another term for menstruation.

Pornography – Magazines, videos, pictures, and printed material designed to stimulate sexual desires.

Pregnant – Having a developing embryo or fetus in the uterus. The average duration of a pregnancy for humans is 280 days or about nine months.

Progesterone – A female sex hormone which is produced by the ovary after ovulation.

Prostrate Gland – A male gland surrounding the urethra at the base of the bladder. It secretes a fluid which is discharged with sperm.

Puberty – A stage in human development when the reproductive organs are becoming mature.

Pubic – The area around the genitals.

Pubic Lice – Annoying tiny creatures that cause intense itching and irritation of the skin, usually around the pubic (genital) area. They are usually spread by sexual intercourse, sexual contact or bed sheets of an infected person. Often referred to as crabs.

Rape – Having penetrative sex with an unwilling person.

Reproductive Organs – The organs which allow men and women to produce children.

Scrotum – A pouch of skin behind the penis which holds the testicles.

Secondary Virginity – The decision to choose a lifestyle of sexual abstinence after a person has already experienced sexual intercourse.

Semen – A milky fluid which transports sperm from the male body.

Sexual Abuse – When a person touches the genital area of an unwilling or unsuspecting person.

Sexual Abuser – Any sexual behavior with an unwilling individual or unsuspecting child. This can include: intercourse; touching of the genitals, breasts, or buttock; exposing to pornography; and offensive sexual talk.

Sexual Arousal – Sexually excited.

Sex Drive – The urge or desire to have sex. A person can choose to control their sex drive or let their sex drive control them.

Sexual Intercourse – Penetration of the penis into the vagina.

Sexually Transmitted Disease (STD) – A disease which is transmitted through sexual intercourse or the skin to skin contact of the genital area. There are 25 significant STDs.

Sperm – Contains the father's hereditary material in 23 chromosomes. When the sperm penetrates the female's egg conception takes place.

Spouse – A marriage partner.

Sterile – Not able to reproduce.

Stillbirth – A child born dead.

Syphilis – A common bacterial sexually transmitted disease. Although this disease can be cured, if left untreated it can lead to death.

Testicles (Testes) – The male reproductive organ which produces testosterone and sperm. Consists of two glands inside the scrotum, located behind the penis.

Testosterone – A male hormone produced by the testicles. It causes male hair growth, rapid muscular and skeletal growth, and development of the penis and testicles which allows men to reproduce.

Tubal Pregnancy – Occurs when a fertilized egg implants in a fallopian tube instead of the uterus. Because the fallopian tube cannot stretch, the tube will rupture, causing hemorrhaging. This can be fatal to the mother. Also known as ectopic pregnancy.

Urethra – A tube which carries urine from the bladder. In females the tube runs from the bladder to the small opening just above the vagina. In the male it runs from the bladder to the end of the penis where urine is eliminated. The male's urethra is also used to deposit semen.

Uterus – A hollow muscular organ in the lower abdomen of a female where a fetus grows and develops for nine months. Also called a womb.

Vagina – The opening between a woman's legs which leads to the uterus. This opening is used for sexual intercourse and is also where a baby passes through at birth.

Venereal Disease (VD) – Another term for sexually transmitted diseases.

Venereal Warts – Warts in the genital or anal area.

Virgin – A male or female who has never had sexual intercourse.

Vulva – The external sexual organs of a female consisting of the labia majora, labia minora, clitoris, and the opening to the vagina and urethra.

Wet Dream – The body's natural way of releasing the build-up of sperm. This happens while a male sleeps and is very normal. Also called "nocturnal emission."

Withdrawal – A method of birth control where the male withdraws the penis before ejaculation occurs. This is not an effective method since small amounts of seminal fluid are released throughout the sexual act. These small drops contain hundreds of thousands of sperm which can still produce a baby.

Womb – A hollow muscular organ in the lower abdomen of a female where a fetus grows and develops for nine months. Also called a uterus.

WORKBOOK ANSWERS

Chapter 1 Pretest

1. B
2. C
3. A
4. A
5. B
6. D
7. A,C,D

Chapter 3

1. A. 1,000
   B. 500 million – to win the race to the females egg
   C. Lower the temperature to protect the sperm
   D. 400
   E. 24 hours
   F. Male's sperm
   G. 5th to 8th
   H. 21st
   I. Young one
   J. 8th
   K. 6
   L. 36 to 40 weeks
2. A. T
   B. F
   C. T
   D. T
   E. F
   F. T
   G. F
   H. F
   I. T

Chapter 6

1. 25
2. 8,219
3. T
4. F
5. Teenage girls
6. Signs, symptoms, contagious
7. T

Chapter 7
1. B
2. D
3. E
4. C
5. A

Chapter 8
1. C
2. A
3. D
4. B
5. A,B,C,D
6. A(for babies),B,C,D

Chapter 10
1. Family member, a friend, a stranger
2. 3
3. 6
4. A. Tries to have a conversation regarding sexual matters
    B. Wants to show you pictures or videos with sexual content
    C. Wants to take seductive pictures or a video of you
    D. Touches you inappropriately
    E. Wants to have sexual intercourse
6. A. Get out of there quickly
    B. Tell your parents or another trusted adult
7. Call the police, clothes, shower, bath, details

Chapter 15
Suggestions to Family Discussion #3.
  A. "Well obviously everyone isn't having sex because I'm not.
      And if you are so convinced everyone's doing it, you shouldn't have
      any trouble finding someone else to do it with."
  B. "If you really love me, how could you ask me to have sex?"
  C. "Hey my dog has sex, and he's not a real man."
  D. "You're going to need protection if you don't keep your hands off me!"

QUICK ORDER FORM

Fax orders: (972) 422-8030   Send this form.

Telephone orders: Call (972) 422-2322   Have your credit card ready.

E-Mail orders: orders@aim-for-success.org

Postal orders: Charles River Publishing Co.
                 P.O. Box 551623
                 Dallas, TX 75355-1623

Please send the following books, audio tapes or CDs. I understand that I may return any of them for a full refund – for any reason, no questions asked.

	Price	Qty	Amount
BOOKS by Marilyn Morris TEENS Sex AND CHOICES	$13.95		
ABC's of the Birds and Bees for Parents of Toddlers to Teens	$17.95		
8 AUDIO TAPES or 3 CDs TEENS Sex AND CHOICES	$24.95		

Please send more FREE information on:

❑ Other material   ❑ Speaking / Seminars

Please PRINT

Name _____

Address_____

City_____ State_____ Zip_____

Telephone (   ) _____

e-mail address _____

Sales Tax: Please add 8.25% if products are shipped to Texas addresses.

Shipping:

U.S.: $4 for the first book, tape or CD and $2 for each additional product. International: $9 for first product and $5 for each additional product.

Payment: ❑ Check   ❑ Credit Card
              ❑ Visa   ❑ MasterCard   ❑ AMEX   ❑ Discover

Card Number: _____

Name on card: _____ Exp Date: /

Signature: _____

QUICK ORDER FORM

Fax orders: (972) 422-8030   Send this form.

Telephone orders: Call (972) 422-2322   Have your credit card ready.

E-Mail orders: orders@aim-for-success.org

Postal orders: Charles River Publishing Co.

                P.O. Box 551623

                Dallas, TX 75355-1623

Please send the following books, audio tapes or CDs. I understand that I may return any of them for a full refund – for any reason, no questions asked.

	Price	Qty	Amount
BOOKS by Marilyn Morris TEENS Sex AND CHOICES	$13.95		
ABC's of the Birds and Bees for Parents of Toddlers to Teens	$17.95		
8 AUDIO TAPES or 3 CDs TEENS Sex AND CHOICES	$24.95		

Please send more FREE information on:

    ❑ Other material   ❑ Speaking / Seminars

Please PRINT

Name _____

Address_____

City _____ State_____ Zip_____

Telephone (_____) _____

e-mail address _____

Sales Tax: Please add 8.25% if products are shipped to Texas addresses.

Shipping:

U.S.: $4 for the first book, tape or CD and $2 for each additional product.

International: $9 for first product and $5 for each additional product.

Payment: ❑ Check   ❑ Credit Card

            ❑ Visa ❑ MasterCard ❑ AMEX ❑ Discover

Card Number: _____

Name on card: _____ Exp Date:____ /____

Signature: _____